I0070928

TCM and You

Just what you need to know about Traditional Chinese Medicine

Clement Ng Shin Kiat

黄欣杰

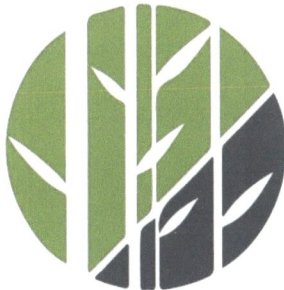

ISBN: 9811163871
ISBN-13: 978-9811163876 (TCM and You)
www.tcmandyou.com

To those who believes that Health is more than Science.

This one's for you.

Contents

Preface

It all began with a request from **Francis Lee,** former President of Raffles Marina, for me to do a series on Traditional Chinese Medicine (TCM) for their club's magazine "Nautique". This book started off as a compilation of the published articles with numerous useful additions, which will be of great use to you. If you believe that Health is more than mere Science, then this book is for you.

My experience teaching executive programs and courses in health and business taught me that a short book on Traditional Chinese Medicine would be useful. I took great effort to distil and condense the key concepts for you that you can grasp TCM and finish this book in half a day.

"TCM and You" captures the essence of just what you'd like to know about Traditional Chinese Medicine. It offers a concise explanation of how TCM, as a medical science and philosophy that has been tested, proven and survive through generations, can play a significant role in addressing the escalating health and medical we are facing today.

"TCM and You" is aimed at individuals who value alternatives in personal health and take ownership in maintaining it. It also contains guidance for health care professionals who help others in their journey towards a healthier lifestyle. This book serves as introductory prerequisite reading for more in-depth sharing on TCM knowledge in my subsequent books.

Chapter one examines the differences between Chinese and Western Medicine. Much debate has surfaced over the differences in Chinese and Western Medicine from the degree of scientific certainty to the availability of evidence-based research and therapeutic treatment approaches. While both exist to help humans who are in constant battle against illnesses, their approaches to diagnosis, treatment and cure are remarkably different. I will address their differences, which will form the basis for the rest of the book.

In Chapter Two, I present what you need to know to restore balance to your life. I share fundamental theories and principles of TCM such as Yin-Yang, Five Elements and how such ancient wisdoms continue to play significant roles in the treatment of illnesses today.

Chapter Three looks at the word "Qi", which is one of the most controversial and misunderstood term for someone new to TCM. As you read through the chapter you will gain a deeper perspective of TCM, appreciate it and articulate it to others whom you think will benefit from TCM.

Chapter Four helps you understand a rise in body temperature, or heatiness from the TCM perspectives. It helps you determine whether reaching out for a cooling drink is a good thing to do when you experience heatiness. This chapter explains how TCM classifies and interprets the relative "heatiness" in our bodies, and their respective symptoms and treatments.

In Chapters Five and Six, I discuss the flow of Qi along our body superhighway, in tandem with the flow generated by forces of nature. Just as our earth is threatened by drastic changes in the global climate, our body can be unbalanced resulting in mood and health changes. I explain the importance of maintaining our internal flow of Qi to ensure that our meridian-collateral system is at its optimal state. I show how TCM identifies and works along this superhighway to keep your body systems in balance, ensuring you stay in the pink of health.

Chapter Seven and Eight complete this selection of insights on "TCM and You" by presenting Body Constitution Differentiation. I guide you through a questionnaire for you to determine your personal body constitution's type and explain how TCM addresses different illnesses and diseases using the syndrome differentiation diagnostic and the concept of body constitution.

Today's escalating cost associated with modern medicine and increasing health issues due to our aging population, knowledge and skill in understanding the options available, and alternative medicines such as TCM is a significant advantage. I strongly believe that the holistic approaches of TCM to diagnosis and treatment hold the keys toward a better healthcare system for generations to come.

It is my goal to make this knowledge easily accessible to those who believe that Health is more than Science.

May the "Qi" be with you!

Clement Ng S. K.

Singapore

February 2018

Acknowledgement

The inspiration from Francis Lee, former President of Raffles Marina, the first Five Gold Anchor rated marinas in the Asia-Pacific region, motivated me to pen my thoughts into concrete words.

The support from Mr Ray Parry, CEO of Raffles Marina, and his Nautique editorial team, in editing and publishing my original articles. In addition, Raffles Marina's Captain Table, helped bring about the fusion of oriental healing into fine culinary art!

The generous contribution of the many photographers from Unsplash.com and Pixabay.com for their high quality pictures, helped make the complex concepts more vivid and lively through touch of creative illustration.

The keen editorial insight of Dr Ng Pan Wei, international acclaimed author and my good friend for making this book more readable and practical.

The creative design and artistic input of Ng Kai Xiang and Ng Kai Rui, my sons, helped introduce originality to the characters illustrated in chapter on the body constitution.

Thank you!

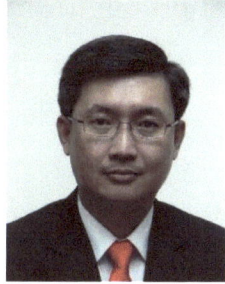

The Author

Dr Clement Ng, is the Principal Consultant, Founder of TCMandYou Pte Ltd and a registered TCM practitioner from Singapore. He is bi-cultural and bilingual in English and Chinese.

Dr Ng is the chairman for the Technical Committee on Complementary Medicine and Health Products in Singapore, in the Biomedical and Health Standards Committee of **"Enterprise Singapore"**. He champions the formulation, recommendation and adoption of standards for TCM, Therapeutic and Complementary Health Product in areas of Manufacturing, Services and Training.

Dr Ng received his Doctorate Degree in Medicine (TCM) from Nanjing University of Chinese Medicine in China and his MBA in Strategic Management from Nanyang Business School, Nanyang Technological University (NTU) in Singapore; he has a Graduate Diploma in Marketing from Chartered Institute of

Marketing, UK, and a Bachelor Degree in Computer Technology from NTU, Singapore.

He provides TCM courses and workshops approved under the Singapore SkillsFuture Training framework. He also shares TCM and Acupressure knowledge on **Udemy,** an online learning and teaching marketplace, reaching out to international students coming from more than 29 countries.

His treatment specialities include Chronic Diabetes Management, Stroke and Paralysis Management, Sleeping Disorders and Eczema /Skin Disorders.

Besides providing professional consultancy, treatment and training services, Dr Ng is the Council Member for Singapore Chinese Physicians' Association, Singapore Acupuncture Association and Representing Singapore as the Expert Committee Member for ISO/TC 249 (TCM) and Executive Council Member for the Specialty Committee for Medicated Diet and Dietotherapy in the World Federation of Chinese Medicine Societies. Dr Ng was the former Vice President of the Singapore College of Traditional Chinese Medicine and the founding Committee member of the Continuous Education Committee for Singapore TCM Practitioner's Board.

Let the health and science journey begins…

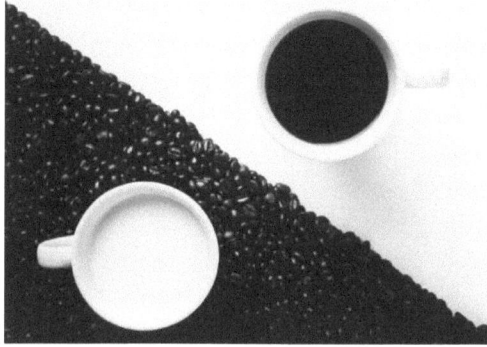

1. Striking A Balance between Traditional and Western Medicine

There has been much debate regarding the differences in Traditional and Western Medicine, covering areas such as their theoretical and scientific basis, the availability of evidence-based researches to validate treatment approaches, and the impact on symptoms and root causes. While both exist to help humans combat against sickness and disease and ensure the survival of civilisation, their approaches to diagnosis, treatment and cure are poles apart.

This chapter will discuss the differences between Chinese and Western Medicine from the perspectives of the understanding of illnesses and diseases, the diagnostic approaches and treatment methodologies.

The Introduction

The adoption of Traditional Chinese Medicine

(TCM) and acupuncture is fast gaining popularity and has been widely touted as a possible answer to the rising medical costs faced by many economies in the 21st century. TCM stands on the shoulders of more than 5,000 years of experience and empirical evidence. Throughout history, the Chinese people have been dependent on Chinese Medicine to cure diseases and to protect themselves against epidemics.

From the over 300 types of traditional medicines practised by different races, TCM has emerged as one that is most systematic and well documented. It includes a wide range of herbal medicines, devices, massage techniques and diets, and has been used as mainstream or alternative medical health systems in over 170 countries. The World Health Organisation (WHO) in 2003, officially endorsed 31 diseases, symptoms or conditions that can be effectively treated using acupuncture, an important form of TCM treatment.

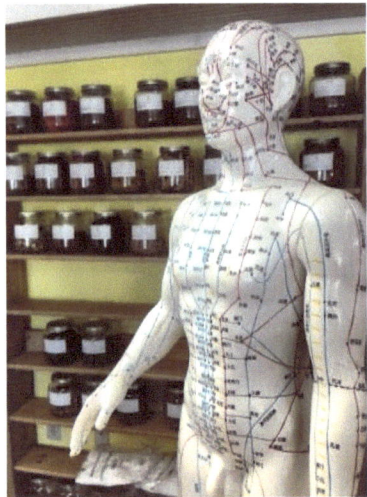

Understanding illnesses and diseases

Before the introduction of Western Medicine to China during the early 19th century by Protestant missionaries, the only medicinal system available in

China was what we know today as TCM. Official records show that it has successfully overcome many diseases and pandemics.

The origins of TCM are deeply rooted in the lives of commoners like you and me. Referencing all Chinese literatures that have survived for generations, we will discover Chinese medicine theories and applications had been widely mentioned, and this further adds to its dimensions and more importantly, its validity. We can find herbal formula and herbal diet cuisine mentioned in Chinese classics such as "A Dream of Red Mansions" (红楼梦) and "Romance of Three Kingdoms" (三国演义). For something that has survived, evolved and developed through thousands of years, it has longitudinal evidence; it is more than science; it is philosophy and is very much an integral part of the Chinese cultures around the world.

Renowned philosophers in China such as LaoZi (老子) and Confucius (孔子) are great practitioners of TCM too. Many of their thoughts on Chinese Medicine that were captured in medical literatures form an integral part of TCM theory today. The state of balance, the key concept

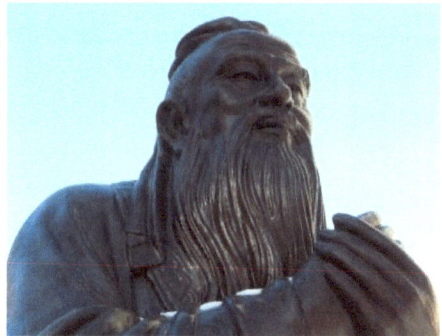

Confucius (孔子)

behind TCM, is a foundation shared by Confucianism and Taoism. Here, all elements are linked and are interdependent on one another; with the concept of yin and yang (阴阳), being a key foundation underlying Taoism.

When western doctors speak of moderation, it is a testimony for the need to stay in balance. The occurrence of illnesses and diseases is the result of an imbalance or the equilibrium between the different elements becoming unstable. TCM adopts a bigger picture and more holistic approach in treating illnesses and diseases. The objective of TCM diagnosis is to discover the cause of imbalance and instability, and through TCM, attempt to bring that "patient" back to a healthy balance and equilibrium state.

From a Western Medicine point of view, the ancient practice of medicine in Greek medical systems mirrored that of TCM, acknowledging that there is art to medicine as well as science, as written in the Hippocratic Oath. However, the "**art**" element has been very much ignored with the discovery of biological treatments, such as antibiotics, along with developments in chemistry, genetics, and lab technology (such as X-ray, MRI etc.). This has led to what we know as modern medicine today, which is more inclined towards scientific evidence. It views

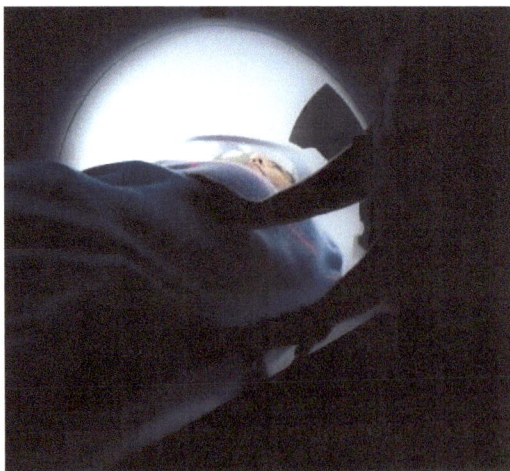

Image on MRI

the occurrence of illnesses and diseases as the result of bacteria or virus attacks or the degeneration of specific organs within the body. Western Medicine adopts a specialized approach diagnosing illnesses and diseases. It requires the identification of the specific bacteria or virus that causes the illness or the degeneration of specific organs or genetic reasons behind the occurrence of the illnesses, before prescribing the necessary medication and treatment protocol for the patient.

Diagnostic Approaches

Western Medicine today relies on many test reports to assist doctors in diagnosing illnesses. While common ailments such as cough, cold, running nose and so on can be easily diagnosed through observation and simple survey-like questions, more complex illnesses and diseases demand lab tests and analysis in order to identify the causes behind illnesses. There are many devices and tools to assist doctors in handling such diagnoses

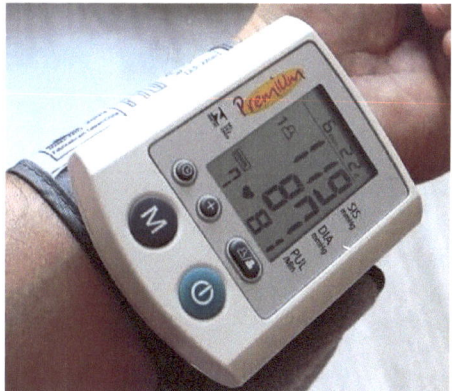

Blood Pressure Meter

as well as home-grade self-diagnostic versions such as thermometers, blood pressure meters and glucometers. Western doctors rely heavily on the readings taken from such devices.

From a Chinese Medicine point of view, the human body is a holistic system that exists in harmony within an environment comprising of social and cultural systems. When an individual and its external environment are not working in harmony, functional impairments will occur with symptoms that include fatigue, numbness, pain, fever and chills. TCM practitioners use a systematic approach of collecting symptoms presented by the patient, a process known as "Syndrome Differentiation", to draw a diagnostic conclusion of the individual's condition and thereby prescribe appropriate treatments.

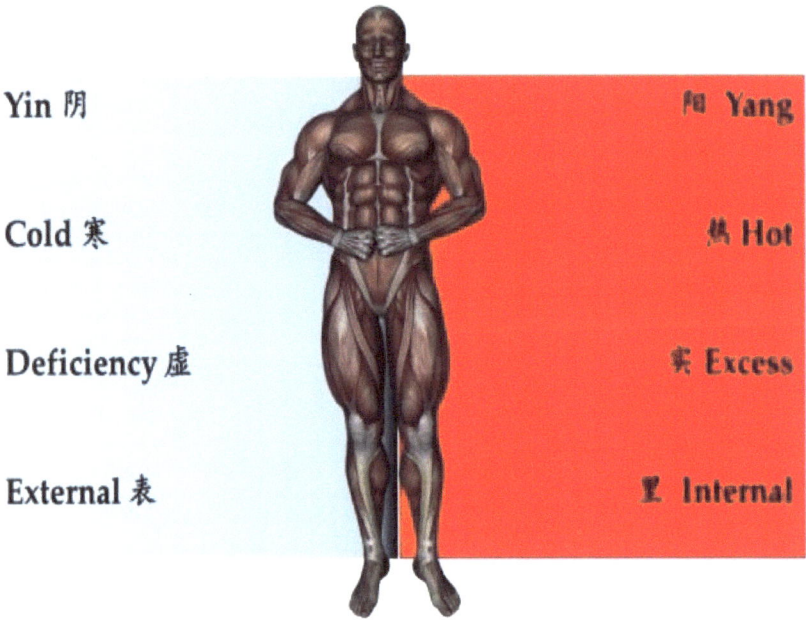

Yin 阴   阳 Yang

Cold 寒   热 Hot

Deficiency 虚   实 Excess

External 表   里 Internal

Syndrome Differentiation Diagnostic

I personally have a strong believe in lab test reports including X-ray and MRI, because they are important medical observations that are very useful for making accurate diagnosis. In my clinical practice, I often request patients to show me their test reports, and at times I will recommend them to get some tests to confirm my diagnosis.

Treatment Methodologies

Diagnostic approaches adopted by western doctor through lab reports and medical device indicators are deemed by western doctors, their patients and other people to be scientific and evidence-base. In contrast, Diagnostic approaches employed by TCM practitioners through syndrome differentiation are not as widely

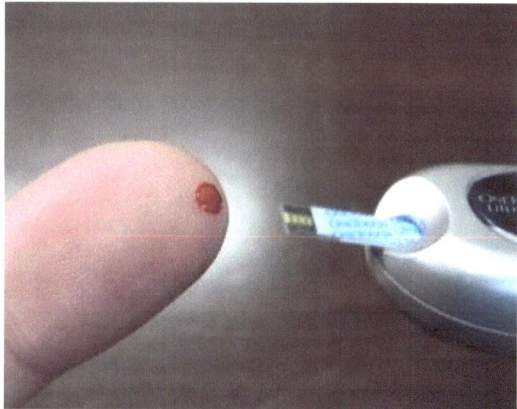
Glucose level monitoring

accepted. Western medicine requires indicators, such as blood pressure readings and glucose levels to guide treatment options that include drugs, physiotherapy and surgery to alleviate symptoms and cure disease. Nevertheless, there will be times when information from reports and the symptoms experienced by patients differ. In such cases, treatment prescribed by their doctors cannot effectively or sufficiently help patients and they continue to suffer the ailments.

WHO (World Health Organisation) define such conditions as being in a state of **Sub-health**; whereby the condition of an individual is between health and disease when all necessary physical and chemical indexes test negative, but the person experiences discomfort or even pain. Western medicine is at its wits' end when dealing with such conditions.

TCM's syndrome differentiating diagnostic approaches are well documented by practitioners over thousands of years and are perfected through generations by legendary physicians such as Hua Tuo (华佗) and Li ShiZhen (李时珍).

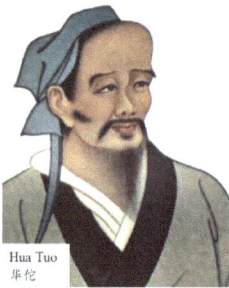

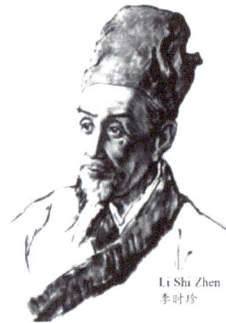

Hua Tuo
华佗

Li Shi Zhen
李时珍

The approach requires TCM practitioners to treat each patient as a unique individual and to draw diagnostic conclusions that are tailored to the patient's syndrome manifestation during the time of consultation, while relying heavily on the practitioner's observation skills and supported by established references and case studies. Patients with the same illness diagnosed by Western doctors will most likely have different TCM prescriptions based on the individual body's constitution and the syndrome presented during consultation. Treatment options include herbal diet, exercise, acupuncture, medicinal herbs and at times, minor surgery.

Such an approach to treatment shows the strength of Chinese Medicine in dealing with sub-health conditions. TCM can play a complementary, if not the main role in preventing further deterioration and maintaining the health of patients who are suffering from pre-chronic or chronic illnesses.

Conclusion

While there are differences in Chinese and Western Medicine as outlined above, both medicinal systems exist with the same objective: To cure patients of illnesses and diseases. The following extract from the Hippocratic Oath applies to both practitioners of Chinese and Western Medicine. **"I will remember that I do not treat a fever chart, a cancerous growth, but a sick human being, whose illness may affect the person's family and economic stability. My responsibility includes these related problems, if I am to care adequately for the sick."**

Statue of Hippocrates

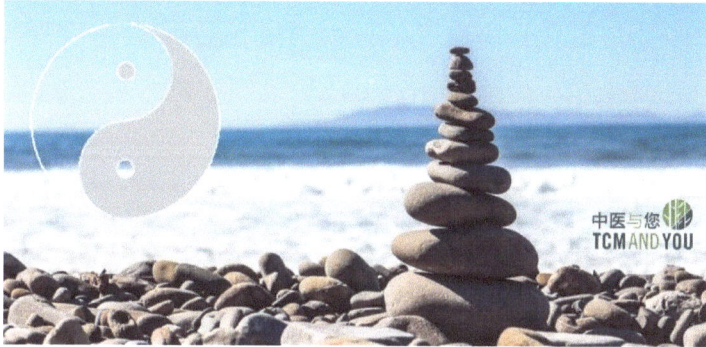

2. Restoring Balance – TCM 101

What is TCM? An ancient art of healing, Traditional Chinese Medicine is a medicinal system that has triumphed over thousands of years of pandemic occurrences and has become an integral part of life for many. Known as Korean Medicine in Korea, Han Medicine in Japan, and Oriental Medicine in America, TCM is based on ancient wisdom passed down from generations in China.

Fundamentals and History

The theory behind TCM was greatly influenced by ancient Chinese materialism and dialectics. The Holism Concept, the Yin-Yang (阴阳) Philosophy and the Five Elements (五行) Theory all descended from ancient Chinese philosophy of interrelated things and phenomena in the natural world; with Treatment By Syndrome Differentiation (TBSD) as distinguishing diagnostic and therapeutic features.

TCM's humble origins include observations on the optimal time to sow, plant, harvest and store our crops, simple pain-relieving massages as well as collective knowledge of therapeutic effects of plants and animals. It accumulated over the centuries as wisdom and experience. TCM has been adopted by over 170 countries today as a viable alternative to conventional western healthcare.

Through the rise and advancement of the Chinese civilization – the invention of paper, the printing press and the sheer hard work of medical practitioners – TCM is continually evolving and is currently one of the most well-documented medicinal systems in the world.

The Holism Concept

Holism has two meanings: Firstly, the equilibrium and harmony of different systems within the human body; secondly, the harmony and close relationship with the external environment in which we are a part of. The human body is composed of various organs along with visceral systems and tissues, each with its own distinct function, but all playing a significant role in our body, all existing in dynamic equilibrium.

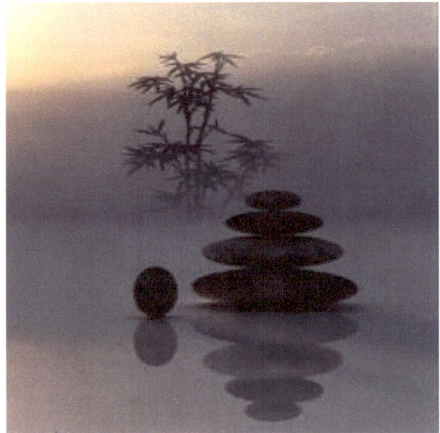

From a TCM perspective, these systems are interrelated and interdependent in physiology, and mutually influential in pathology. As part of the universe; we are affected directly or indirectly by the changes in nature..

A good TCM practitioner has to know the law of nature and geographical conditions when diagnosing and treating diseases. People from different parts of the world exhibit different kinds of illness patterns. This is why TCM not only stresses the unity of the human body itself, but also attaches great importance to the interrelationship between body and nature in diagnosing and treating diseases.

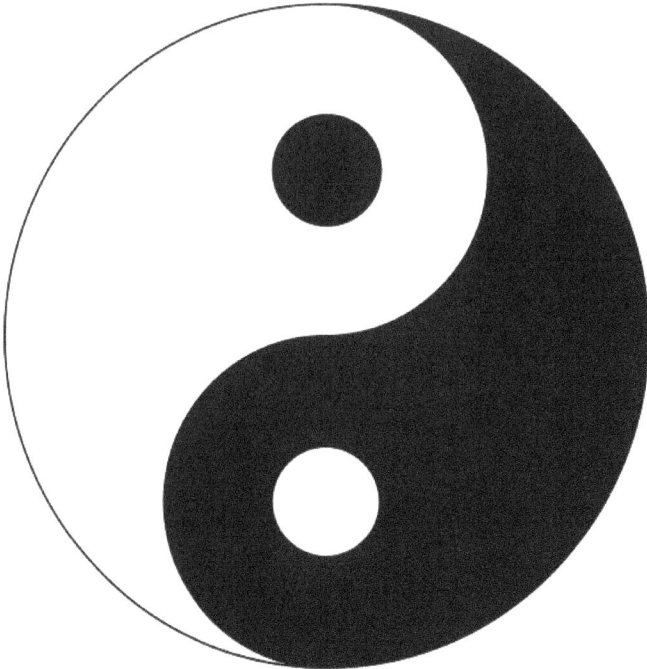

The Taiji Diagram

The Yin-Yang Philosophy ~ The Law Of Nature

The origins of yin-yang can be traced to the Book of Change or I-Jing (易 经), an ancient Chinese philosophy. It is a general term for two opposites of interrelated things or phenomena in the natural world.

By observing the relationship between the moon and the sun, and their impact on the seasons, this philosophy has developed into a relational theory, which may have direct influence on the development of the principle of relativity by Albert Einstein.

In TCM, "everything in the universe contains Yin and Yang". The theory not only represents two opposite objects, but also analyses two opposite aspects existing within every single entity. It holds that the development and changes of everything in the universe that results from the unity of opposites - Yin and Yang. It is used to explain the physiology and pathology of the body and to guide clinical diagnosis and treatment.

The Five Elements Theory

In ancient times, the Chinese believed that all things in nature could be attributed to one of the five elements. This includes the human body, which allows TCM practitioners to diagnose and prescribe appropriate treatments for their patients. Let us explore the classification of things in nature and in turn, the five elements.

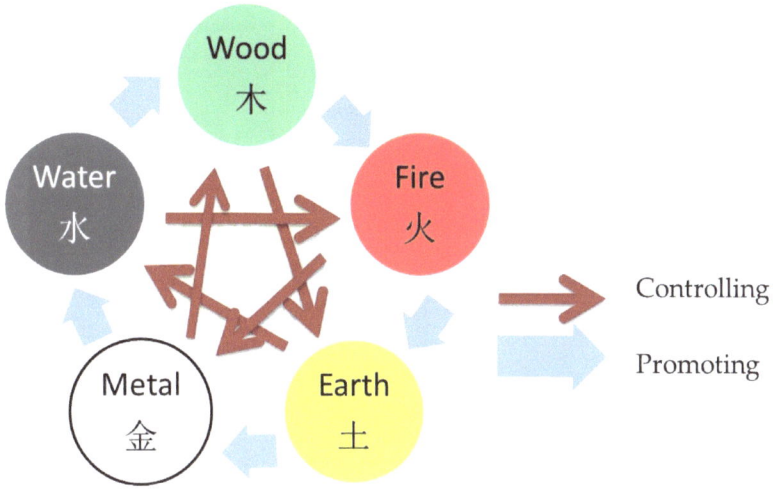

The Five Element Flows

Wood has the nature of growing freely and unfolding. Things that have similar characteristics fall within the wood element. This corresponding analogy continues with the other elements. Fire has the nature of flaring up. Earth has the nature of giving birth to all things. Metal has the nature of purifying and descending. Water has the nature of moistening and flowing downwards.

There are inter-relationships among the five elements; when one element generates, another one will control. These help practitioners diagnose and treat patients.

The following table associates things in nature and their classification according to the 5 elements.

	Wood	Fire	Earth	Metal	Water
Zang	Liver	Heart	Spleen	Lung	Kidney
Fu	Gall bladder	Small intestine	Stomach	Large intestine	Urinary bladder
Senses	Eye	Tongue	Mouth	Nose	Ear
Flavours	Sour	Bitter	Sweet	Pungent	Salty
Tissue	Tendon	Vessel	Muscle	Hair/ skin	Bone
Directions	East	South	Centre	West	North
Changes	Germinate	Grow	Transform	Reap	Store
Colour	Green	Red	Yellow	White	Black

5 Elements Classification Table

To generate implies that one element can promote aid or bring forth another, e.g. wood generates fire, fire generates earth, earth generates metal, metal generates water; and water, in turn, generates wood. Each of the five elements contains the dual nature of "being generated" and "generating".

To control means restraint, i.e. wood restricts earth, earth does water, water does fire, fire does metal, and metal, in turn, does wood. Any one of the five elements has two aspects, being controlled and controlling others. For example, the element controlling wood is metal, and the element that is controlled by wood is earth.

The five elements oppose yet complement each other. Without generation, there will be no growth and development of things; without the counter effect of control, there will be no balance and coordination during developments and changes. So, how does this theory relate to our body? TCM practitioners observe external symptoms manifested by patients to identify any abnormal changes of the internal organ visceral systems' functions and inter-relationships.

Changes in a patient's skin complexion colour, sense of taste or pulse reflects the corresponding systems within the same element and can be used to diagnose disease. Take for example:

- when a patient is presented with a flushed red face, accompanied by a bitter taste in the mouth and a forceful pulse, these external appearances may point to a heart visceral system disease related to heatiness;

- a person who looks dull and yellowish in complexion and with an appetite for all things sweet may imply that the spleen visceral system is deficient ;

- someone whose complexion has turned darker may imply that the kidney visceral system is deficient;

- if a patient is observed to have a green hue in his complexion, a sour taste in his mouth, and his eyes are bothersome to him in some way, we would look toward the liver visceral systems for further diagnosis;

- when a patient is having a running nose with a pale-white complexion we would possibly associate him with lung visceral system vitality deficiency.

The Five element theory is also useful in the areas of disease prognosis, development and prevention. The progression and prevention of diseases is intricately related to the mutual relationship of generation and control. One classical TCM text, the Nanjing (难经), says, "When the liver visceral systems is diseased, the liver visceral systems symptoms will eventually transmit to the spleen visceral systems, and so one should replenish the system vitality of the spleen visceral systems while considering the treatment protocol for the liver visceral systems." This reflects the clinical application of five element's controlling theory.

Conclusion

From the TCM perspective, the natural world and life processes are full of vitality because there are checks and balances between the different elements, the dynamic equilibrium between Yin and Yang, and holism. The occurrence of a disease or illness signifies a breakdown of dynamic equilibriums and corresponding syndromes will be manifested. During consultation, TCM practitioners determine syndromes by observing elements manifested by the individual. Thereafter, TCM practitioners will diagnose and prescribe the necessary treatment, with **the objective of restoring balance and bringing the individual back to equilibrium.**

Health = Balance

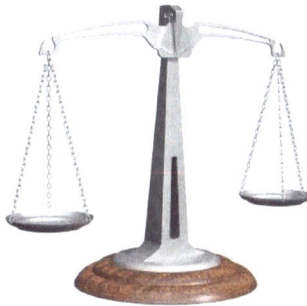

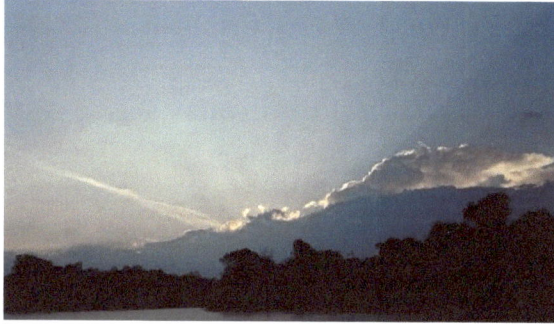

3. May The "Qi" Be With You!

The word **Qi** 气 (pronounced "chee") has been one of the most controversial and misunderstood word for people who may not have a full understanding of TCM. As we journey through this book, I believe you will gain a deeper perspective of TCM， appreciate it and articulate it to others whom you think will benefit from TCM.

By observing the elements in our natural environment and understanding their theoretical applications, TCM has evolved over the generations and has perfected into a systematic diagnosis approach for TCM practitioners today. The concept of Qi, similarly, has been an integral component of these oriental philosophies and forms part of the evolution intricate to the cultural fabric of the Chinese civilisation.

Philosophical aspect of Qi

The original calligraphic symbol of Qi found in

the Oracle (甲骨文) was 3 straight lines ☰ , which means free flowing substance occurring in the natural environment, the force which fills the universe, and the energy behind the continuous movement of elements. It evolved into curly lines 气 which represent the different direction of flow of the elements (Air, water, etc.) and subsequently into the traditional Chinese word form of Qi 氣, which is made up of 气 (a simpler symbol of Qi) and 米 (rice, representing food substance) suggesting that the transformation and production of Qi from food substances. The word is later further simplified into what we know today as Qi 气.

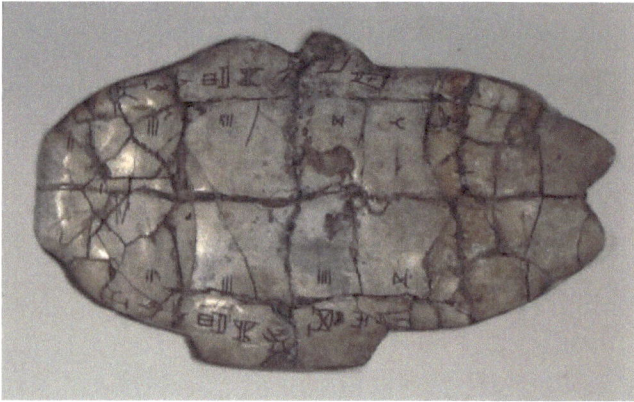

Oracle (甲骨文)

From the philosophical perspective, there exists a trinity Qi relationship between the 3 pillars of the universe: **Heaven** (天"Tian"), **Human** (人"Ren") and **Earth** (地"Di"). It is only when this trinity relationship is in balance from the holistic theory that lifeform on earth will be in abundance and equilibrium.

Heaven Qi is most important, consisting of forces such as sunshine, moonlight, gravity and energy from the stars and planets. Earth Qi is regulated by Heaven Qi and according to Chinese theory, it is made up of lines and patterns of energy, the earth's magnetic field and underground heat provides abundant supply for all things on Earth to survive.

Each person has their own internal Qi which always seeks to achieve balance. As such, besides TCM, the word Qi has permeated into all parts of Chinese culture and language where we use it to explain the vitality of the energy as well as the functionality of elements. Such as

- 生气 (Angry – a burst of energy),
- 天气 (Weather – the nature of the environment),
- 勇气 (Courage – the ability to fight or defend),
- 气质 (Temperament – a person's natural behaviour),
- 气候 (Climate – the prevailing weather conditions),
- 小气 (Stingy – the inability to give),
- 大气层 (The atmosphere), etc.

Besides being used to help to explain the energetic substance or "life force" circulating through the human body and actuating on body's motions, **Qi** is also used to explain the functionality and vitality of different organ visceral systems.

Qi is also seen as the root of life. The first comprehensive TCM medical book was written in 475BC, Huangdi's Inner Classic of Medicine（黄帝内经.） It stated that "The gathering of qi produces life while the dispersion of qi puts an end to life."（气聚则生、气散则亡）. The Qi concept is used in this book to detail human physiological functions and pathological changes, and provides guidance to the diagnosis and prevention of diseases in TCM.

Sources and Types of Qi

According to TCM, there are two major sources of Qi within the human body. The **Congenital Qi** (Prenatal or Innate Essence Qi) exists right after the formation of an individual's life. This kind of Qi - inherited from our parents - is the foundation of the development of new life. After birth, the human body absorbs nutrients from the external world to nourish the Congenital Qi. This is known as **Acquired Qi** (Post-natal Qi), which is the Qi that we generate within our lifetime from the air that we inhale, and the food that we eat. Thus, if one is not blessed with a good Congenital Qi, one can always attain healthy body through Acquired Qi.

To help in the diagnosis and determination of the states of heath of an individual, TCM further classifies Qi into the following types.

- The **Primordial Qi** (Yuan Qi 元气), also known as genuine qi (Zheng Qi 正气) is the most important of the four kinds of Qi. It is the primary drawing force of one's life activities. When someone is seriously injured, we use the Chinese idiom "元气大伤" (Yuan Qi Da Shang) to describe his dire state of health.

- The **Pectoral Qi** (Zong Qi 宗气), is a combination of the fresh air we inhale and the food we eat. The Pectoral Qi travels through the respiratory tract to promote respiration and influences the quality of one's voice, speech and breathing. Thus when someone is unable to project his voice, we use the Chinese idiom "宗气不足" (Zong Qi Bu Zu) to explain his state of health.

- The **Nutritive Qi** (Ying Qi 营气), is the qi that circulates together with blood through the vessels of our bodies. The Nutritive Qi is responsible for blood production and nutrition for the whole body. When we see someone who is undernourished, we use the statement "营养不良" (Ying Yang Bu Liang) to describe his situation.

- The **Defensive Qi** (Wei Qi 卫气), provides a perimeter defence around the body surface to guard against exogenous pathogens. It controls the opening and closing of the pores, and adjusts the excretion of sweat, and maintains a relatively constant body temperature. A person who perspires easily is deem to be weak in Defensive Qi, or "卫气虚" (Wei Qi Xu)

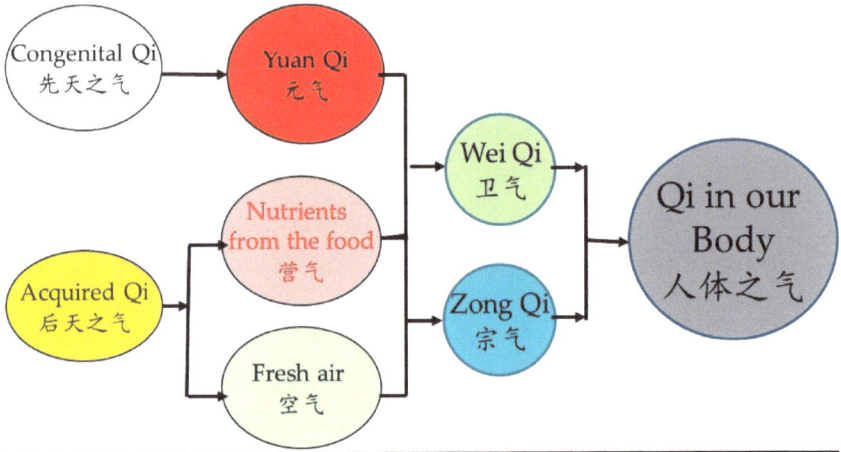

The Family of Qi within the body

Qi, like natural elements in the universe and the free flowing air around us, is constantly active and circulating in living human bodies; it is the "life force" that allows all human activities to take place. Such movement of Qi in the body is known as Qi dynamics "气机", which refers to the Ascending, Descending, Expelling and Absorbing actions of Qi related to the organ visceral system functions. A TCM practitioner will observe the manifestations of Qi disorders presented by the patient to determine the nature of his illness.

Disorders of Qi

The disorders of Qi occur when an individual is experiencing either a deficiency in Qi or a disturbance to the regular flow of Qi. Qi deficiency in the body is typically caused by an inadequate production of Qi due to malnutrition or when Qi is quickly depleted due to lack of rest, which manifests itself through deficiency syndromes and hypo-functions of visceral systems.

A disturbance of Qi such as **Qi Stagnation** （气滞）, occur when the movement of Qi is blocked or does not flow normally. Typical syndromes of Pain pain and swelling in an organ are examples of stagnant Qi.

A **Qi Reversal** （气逆）, occurs when the Qi does not flow according to visceral system Qi dynamics. Manifestations of this condition include vomiting which occurs when the stomach Qi, which is supposed to help in food digestion, reverses its Qi flow.

A situation of Qi **Prolapse** （气陷）occur when the body is not able to perform its function of holding or supporting the organ visceral systems in the right place. Manifestation of this condition include uterus prolapse in women, and hernia in men.

Balanced Qi dynamics in the human body help to maintain normal physiological activities. When the equilibrium of the Qi is disturbed, such as when there is a blockage in the Qi flow, it will result in a steep increase in the levels of Qi and such pent-up Qi which will lead to illnesses.

Regulation of Qi

As quoted in Huangdi's Inner Classic of Medicine （黄帝内经）, "The gathering of Qi produces life while the dispersion of Qi puts an end to life."

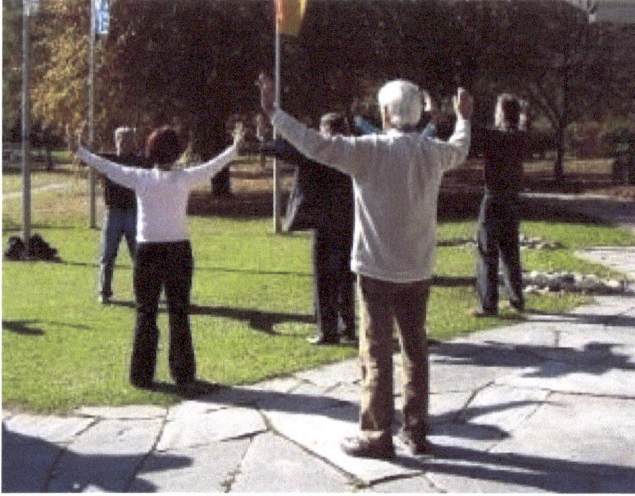

Qigong Practice

TCM adopts different approaches to regulate Qi within our body. Qigong practice is one of the more common approaches and it conditions our bodies to be in harmony with the universe. Qigong is an ancient art form to strengthen the body's vital energy. It works to shorten illness recovery time, improve energy levels, and immune function, hence restore balance in our body using a variety of methods.

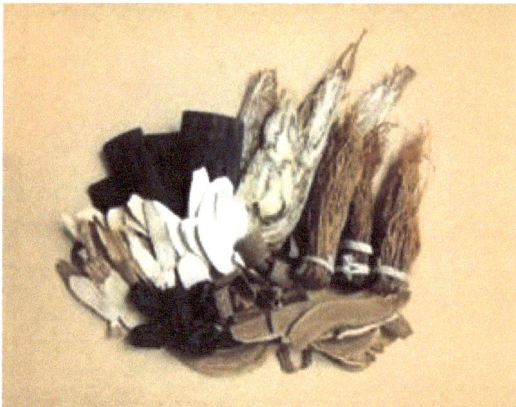

Herbs use in Medicated Diet

Besides Qigong, herbs medicine and medicated diets are used by TCM both to invigorate and energize Qi deficiencies and to move Qi around the body. to avoid stagnation.

Herbs that invigorate and energize Qi include Ren Shen, Dang Shen, Huang Qi, Shan Yao , Bai Zhu, and Hong Zao,.

Herbs to regulate Qi stagnation include Chen Pi, Zhi Shi, Xiang Fu, Mu Xiang, Tan Xiong (sandalwood, Santalum album), and Mei Gui Hua (Rosa rugosa).

May the "Qi" be with you !

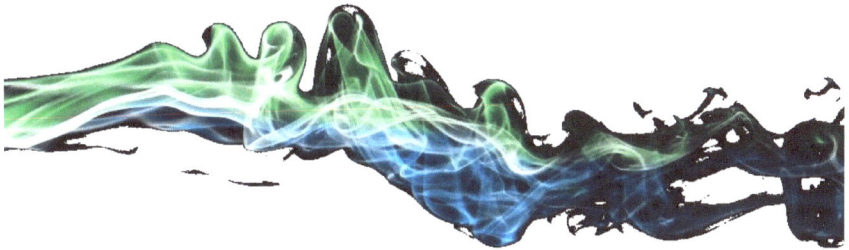

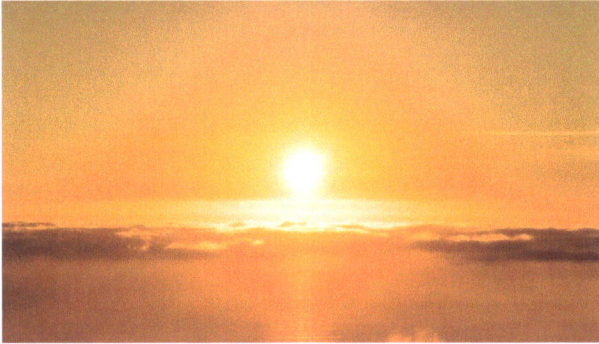

4. Are You "Hot" or Not?

For those in Singapore, living so near the equator and having a tropical rainforest climate to boot makes most of our days warm and humid, which makes many of us feel hot and bothered. We instinctively reach out for that cooling drink (chrysanthemum tea or "Liang-Teh" in local dialect) in a bid to cool down and relieve our that heaty feeling. Yet, is this "heatiness" really attributed to external temperatures, or is there an underlying state of nutritional deficiency within our bodies that need to be addressed.

What is Hot?

Hot is defined as having a high degree of heat or a high temperature. Heat can be defined as a measure of warmth or coldness of an object or substance with reference to some standard value. From the perspective of a human body, heatiness is a sense of the body feeling warm. This symptom has become one of the key observations, which both modern and TCM medicinal practitioners use, to determine whether a person is suffering from an illness.

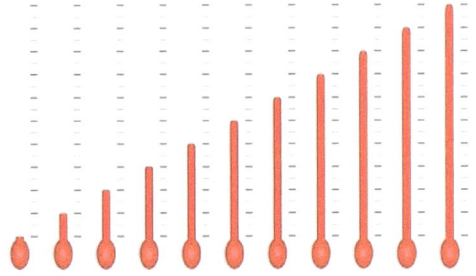

From a TCM perspective, heat has a dual effect in the human body. It is the source of energy for all activities in the body and is responsible for an effective rate of metabolism. TCM practitioners use it to classify syndromes associated with Yin and Yang imbalance, when conducting a "Syndrome Differentiation" diagnostic analysis. A healthy individual cannot survive without heat; but at the same time, too much heat is undesirable. It is the universal goal of TCM treatment to correct imbalance and restore harmony of the body.

Relative Heat?

As discussed in the previous chapter, TCM believes that all substances and energies in the body strive to achieve constant balance and equilibrium relative to one another, in order to sustain health and vitality of the body. This balance is expounded by the **"Yin-Yang Theory"** which forms a basic guideline of the TCM holistic approach.

The transformation between Yin and Yang occurs in a natural and seamless fashion when we are in balance. As you can observe in the Yin-Yang symbol of the Tai-Ji Diagram, you'll see the largest part of the black Yin's ball starting to flip over into the smallest part of the white Yang's tail, and vice versa, as one changes into the other.

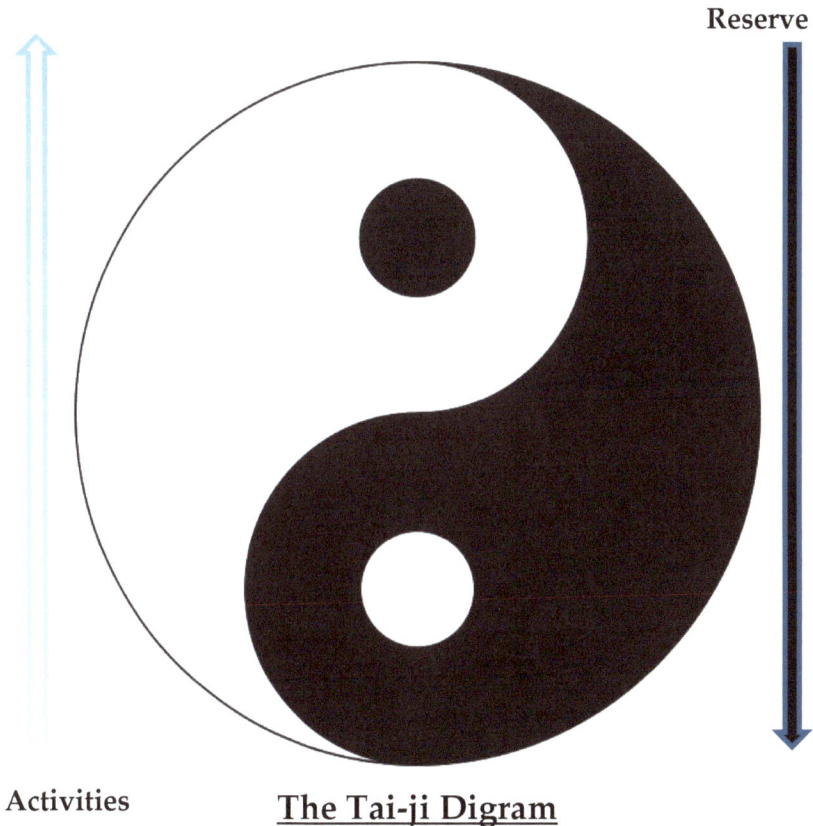

Reserve

Activities

The Tai-ji Digram

Such transformation can be observed in our body energy levels as we go through the day. In the morning, when activities are low - the ascending white arrow -

we are full of reserve and do not feel tired; as the day progresses, activities pick up and reserves are depleted. In the evening, as the activities reached its peak and starts to decline, reserves will start to build up - the descending black arrow - in preparation for next day. Such cycle of energy levels occur naturally.

In the dynamic equilibrium state, Yin (substances or reserves) must stay in balance with Yang (actions or activities), visceral organ systems must work harmoniously in unison, and Shen (emotions) must stay calm for true well-being. This can be achieved through an observed routine and regime of rest, work and regular diet.

However, as we journey through life, with all the activities presented to us in our modern lifestyles, such a dynamic balance is difficult to sustain. Moreover as we age, we will start to experience syndromes, which are associated with imbalance between our Yin and Yang. When this imbalance occurs, individuals will experience symptoms with different degree and nature of "heatiness".

Let me illustrate this development of heatiness brought on by our lifestyle. In "Picture: Yin – Yang" Balance, you will notice that both the Yin and Yang columns align with one another at the balance line. This is an equilibrium state.

阳 Yang   阴 Yin

平衡
Balance

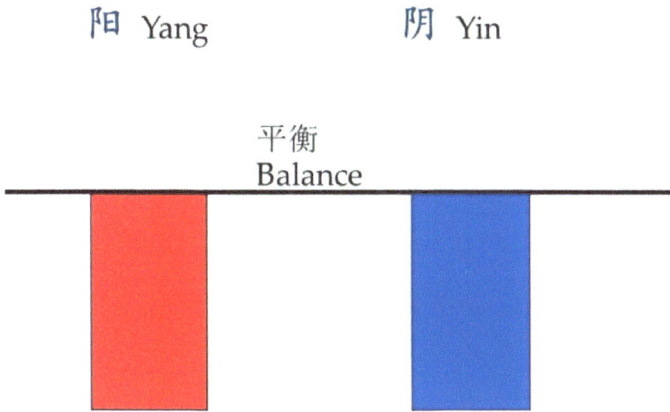

Picture : Yin – Yang Balance

When an individual consumes spicy and oily foods such as curry mutton and fried chicken, the scenario in "Picture: Yang Excess" will take place. One will feel "heatiness" due to an absolute excess of Yang, and will manifest symptoms such as redness in the face, extreme restlessness, agitation, a thirst for cold beverages, a dry mouth and throat, hotness all over the body throughout the day, and a rapid and full pulse.

阳 Yang   阴 Yin

阳甚而热
Yang Excess - heatiness

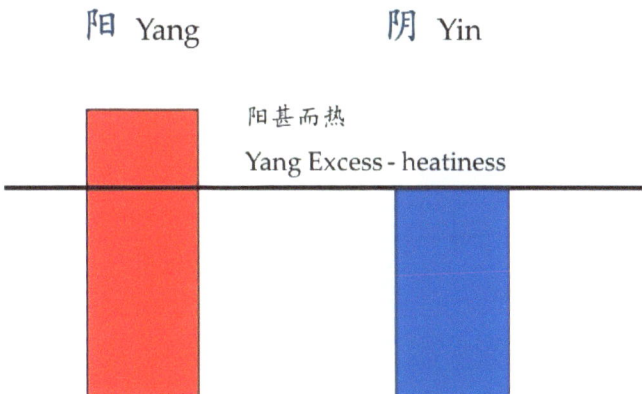

Picture: Yang Excess

When an individual stays up late over many nights, a scenario such as "Picture: Yin Deficiency" will be observed. One will feel "heatiness" due to yin deficiency, a situation when the body's reserves are depleted below the balance line. Symptoms displayed include red or malar hot flush, an emotional state of restlessness, tired and fidgety, a dry mouth and throat at night, mild heat sensation mainly in the afternoon or evening, red line inside eyelid, and a rapid and thin pulse.

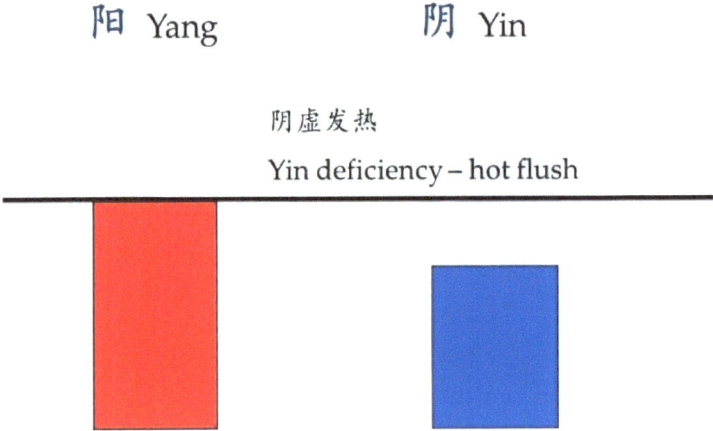

阳 Yang   阴 Yin

阴虚发热
Yin deficiency – hot flush

Picture: Yin Deficiency

Symptoms of heatiness

Comparison of Yin Deficiency and Yang Excess		
	Yin Deficiency	**Yang Excess**
Hotness	Relative	Absolute
Complexion	Red cheeks/malar flush	Whole face red

36

Mental state	Mentally restless but tired, vague anxiety, fidgety	Extreme restlessness, agitation or manic behaviour
Sleep pattern	Frequent waking during night	Dream-disturbed or restless sleep
Thirst	Thirsty, with no desire to drink	Thirst for cold beverages
Mouth	Dry mouth and throat at night	Constant dry mouth and throat
Bowel	Dry stools, no pain	Constipation, pain
Eyes	Red line inside eyelid	Red eyes
Tongue	Red with little coating, or peeled	Red with yellow coating
Pulse	Rapid, thin	Rapid, full

Yin-Yang in Men and Women

It was also observed and documented in the TCM classic text Huangdi's Inner Classic of Medicine (黄帝内经), that as we age, we will naturally start to have low gender-related Yin or Yang energy.

For example, women's Yin decline as they go through menopause. Yin deficiency symptoms include hot flushes, night sweats and frequent night-time waking. Some will grow less submissive, that is, going out, doing more and standing up for themselves. If the situation becomes pathological, they may become restless, easily agitated and more demanding. This is all relative to one's personal observation or proximity to the individual.

Men's Yang decreases as they mellow with age. They become more Yin, that is, easy going, less confrontational and less combative. Yang deficiency symptoms include sexual impotence (enter the multi-billion dollar market for aphrodisiac supplements), frequent waking at night to go to the bathroom, feeling cold and lower back pain. If the situation becomes pathological, they may become too mellow, to the point of losing confidence, becoming listless and apathetic.

The following picture outlines the changes,

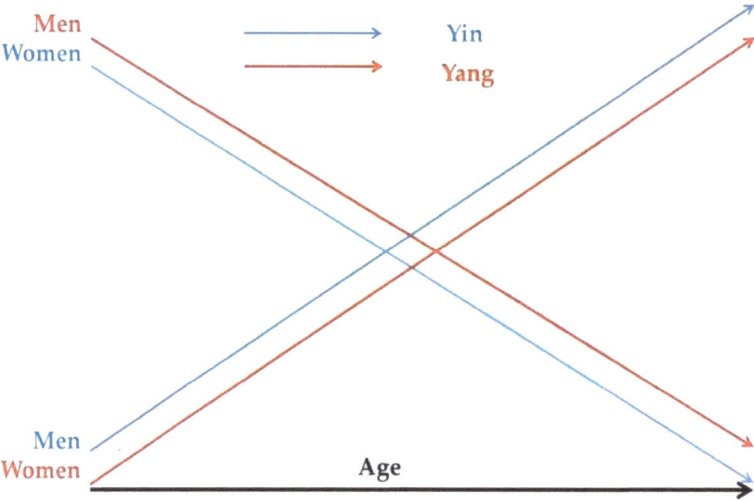

Changes of Yin-Yang in Men and Women with age

Treatment for Heatiness

From what we've learnt so far heat causes restlessness. However, there exists differences in whether the heatiness is due to Yin deficiency or Yang-excess. A Yin-deficient individual will experience inexplicit anxiety without the ability to pinpoint why and what causes this edginess. A Yang-excess individual is obviously more agitated, and sometimes arrogant; and any heaty sensation will cause difficulties in falling and staying asleep. Even if sleep comes, the person is extremely restless and full of dreams. But a Yin-deficiency heatiness keeps people waking frequently during the night or early morning.

A correct diagnostic and appropriate treatment protocol needs to be administered to correct such imbalance and resume harmony within the body. In general, we nourish Yin when there is Yin deficiency, and clear heat when there is an excess of it. However, in the event of a misdiagnosis or the individual decides to self-medicate with limited knowledge, the following scenarios will occur.

In "Picture: Damp heatiness", instead of clearing the heat during a Yang-excess situation, Yin-nourishing treatment was administered. For example, instead of consuming cooling tea like chrysanthemum tea, one chooses to drink a soup prepared with an ingredient such as Polygonatum Odoratum （玉竹: yuzhu）which is typically used for nourishing the Yin. A situation of damp-heatiness will occur.

阳 Yang   阴 Yin

湿热
Damp
heatiness

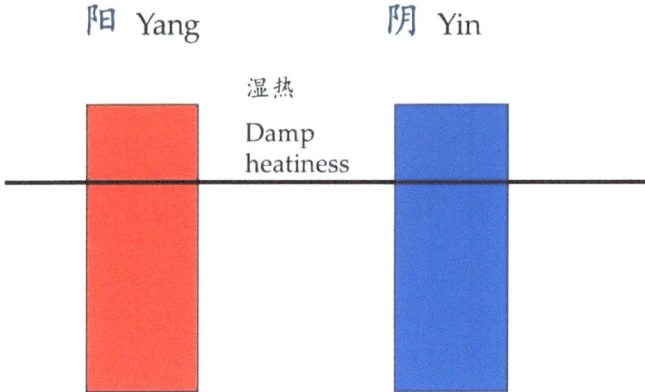

Picture: Damp heatiness

On the other hand, to nourish Yin deficiency due to over exertion and age-related scenarios, we adopt a purging protocol instead of nourishing Yin, a situation in "Picture 5: Weaken Body" will occur. While the individual may feel relieve from the reduction of heatiness, such mistreatment actually results in a weaker body constitution, which is undesirable in the long run.

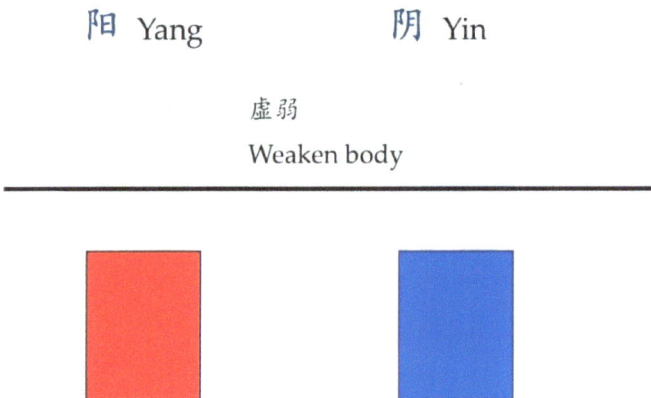

阳 Yang   阴 Yin

虚弱
Weaken body

Picture 5: Weaken Body

From a TCM perspective, there are five common types of Yin deficiencies, and three types of Yang excesses, all of which result in different degrees of heatiness. The objective of this chapter is to let you familiarise with the general symptoms associated with heatiness.

So, next time when you experience heatiness, while it is alright to reach out for your favourite cooling beverage, you may want to go a little deeper to address the underlying state of your body.

Are you hot or not?

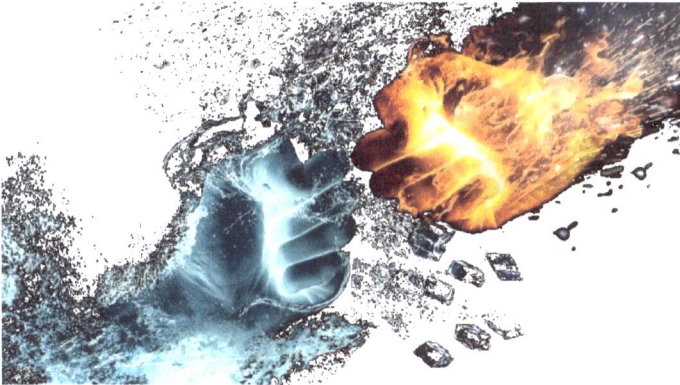

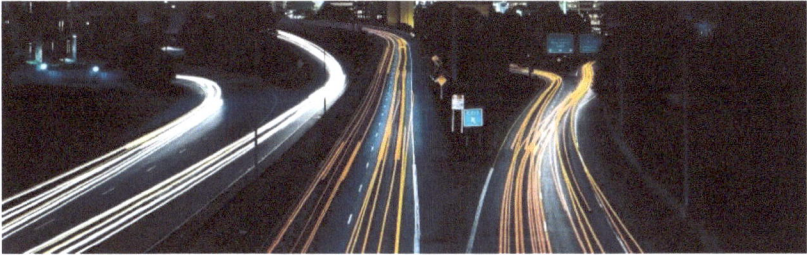

5. The Body Super Highway

The flow of Qi along our body superhighway move in a defined direction with a continuous even flow generated by forces of nature. Just as the universe is threatened by drastic changes in global climate, our body can lose balance resulting in mood and health changes. In this chapter, I will explain the importance of maintaining our Qi's internal flow and ensure that our health retains its optimal state.

For those who love the sea and enjoy sailing or any sea sport, I believe you will be familiar with wind, weather, and ocean conditions when you set sail for the open sea. Ocean currents move in a continuous direction generated by forces acting upon the seawater; creating breaking waves, winds, the Coriolis Effect, temperature and salinity differences. Meanwhile, tides are caused by the gravitational pull of the sun and moon, the Yang and the Yin. (for an animated map of the current wind, weather, ocean, visit https://earth.nullschool.net/)

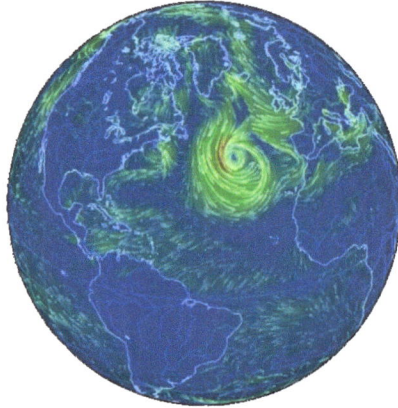

Source: https://earth.nullschool.net

A major tenet of TCM is the belief that humans are part of the universe and there exists an internal universe within us that always strives to achieve a balance and harmony with the external. TCM founders base their observations on natural phenomena to derive and apply concepts such as the Five Elements in their understanding of the human body. Drawing upon their observations of the ocean current – the movement of winds in continuous and directed movement in a periodic pattern, influencing weather conditions – they postulated the existence of an energy

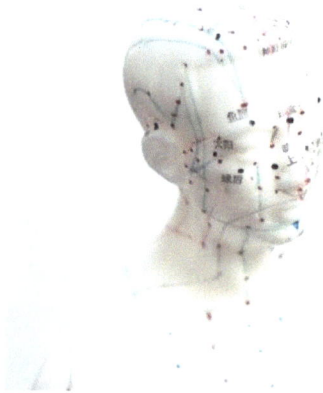

or Qi movement in our body that is also continuous, directed and periodic movement.

We call this movement of Qi in our bodies the **Meridian-Collateral system** – it's your body's Qi superhighway! Just like ocean currents – which can be categorised into surface oceanic currents, deep oceanic currents, south equatorial currents of the Atlantic, horizontal and vertical currents – the meridian-collateral systems of the body also have their corresponding nomenclature which are named after the body's visceral systems as well as the nature of their respective meridians.

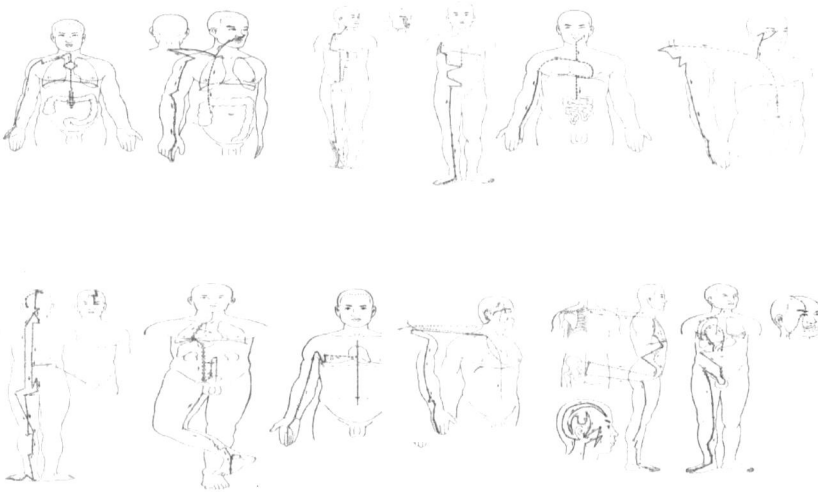

The 12 Primary Meridians' Pathway

For those who reside in Southeast Asian countries such as Singapore and Malaysia, you will notice that every year during July to September, a grey hue will overshadow the clear sky, as the South-West Monsoon channels the haze created by the ever-burning peat fire from Indonesia. Just like the Seasonal Monsoon Wind Systems, with its fixed timing and predictable path, acting on global climatic behaviours and corresponding agricultural activities, the Meridian-Collateral system in our body traverse in fixed timings and predictable paths acting on the health of an individual and the corresponding health maintenance activities.

The Meridian - Collateral System network in our body is divided into two categories: the JingMai (经脉) or meridian channels system, and the LuoMai (络脉) or the collaterals system. The meridian channels system is the main distribution pathway for Qi or energy throughout the body through the 12 principal meridians, the eight extraordinary meridians and the collateral system.

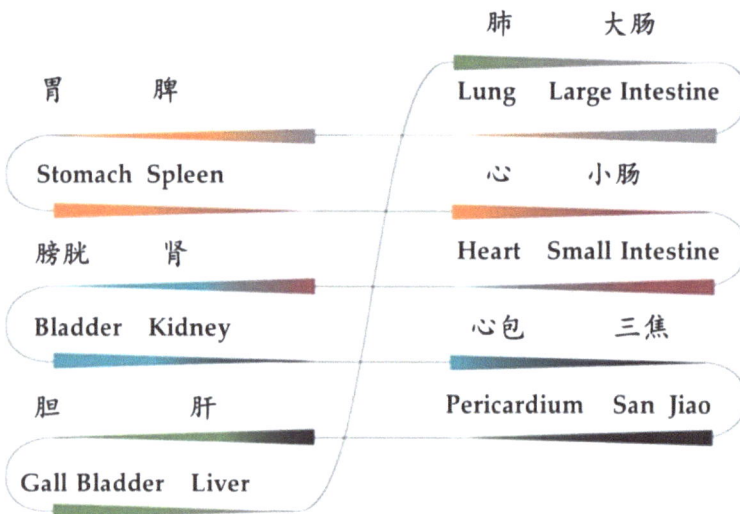

肺　　大肠

胃　　脾

Lung　Large Intestine

Stomach　Spleen

心　　小肠

膀胱　　肾

Heart　Small Intestine

Bladder　Kidney

心包　　三焦

胆　　肝

Pericardium　San Jiao

Gall Bladder　Liver

The 12 Primary Meridians Flow Sequence

The meridian channels system connects to the 12 principal meridians in various ways – through the visceral systems of internal organs and other related internal structures. If one counts the number of unique points on each meridian, the total comes to 361, which incidentally is the number of days in a lunar calendar year.

The 12 principal meridians are divided into Yin and Yang groups. Yin meridians in the arm run through the lung, heart, and pericardium. Yang meridians in the arm consist of the Large Intestine, Small Intestine, and San Jiao. Yin meridians in the leg are the Spleen, Kidney, and Liver. Yang meridians in the leg are Stomach, Bladder, and Gall Bladder. These 12 principal meridians are symmetrical on the right and left sides of the body, and are all interconnected with each other.

The Flowing Order of The 12 Principal Meridians

Qi is the material basis and energy for our bodies' life activities. Just as ocean currents serve as conveyor belts transporting warm water from the equator to the poles, and cold water from the poles back to the tropics, Qi uses the body's Meridian-Collateral System to transport and distribute itself throughout the body. It warms, nourishes and moistens all organ visceral systems and tissues, and maintains normal functions of the body.

Qi within the 12 primary meridians traverse their corresponding organ visceral systems, circulating the body in a never-ending loop throughout our lives. Their circulation starts from the lung meridian of hand-Taiyin and runs to the liver meridian, following a time-period analogy to the Chinese zodiac calendar as well as traditional time references. Each meridian is associated with their corresponding time-period of the day, which plays a significant and practical role in TCM health maintenance routines.

Time of Day (Chinese)			Organ Visceral (Chinese)	Meridian name (Chinese)
23:00 - 1:00	zǐ shí	子時	Gall Bladder (胆)	Shaoyang Gallbladder Meridian of Foot (足少阳胆经)
1:00 - 3:00	chǒu shí	丑時	Liver (肝)	Jueyin Liver Meridian of Foot (足厥阴肝经)
3:00 - 5:00	yín shí	寅時	Lung (肺)	Taiyin Lung Meridian of Hand (手太阴肺经)
5:00 - 7:00	mǎo shí	卯時	Large Intestine (大肠)	Yangming Large Intestine Meridian of Hand (手阳明大肠经)
7:00 - 9:00	chén shí	辰時	Stomach (胃)	Yangming Stomach Meridian of Foot (足阳明胃经)
9:00 - 11:00	sì shí	巳時	Spleen (脾)	Taiyin Spleen Meridian of Foot (足太阴脾经)
11:00 - 13:00	wǔ shí	午時	Heart (心)	Shaoyin Heart Meridianof Hand (手少阴心经)
13:00 - 15:00	wèi shí	未時	Small Intestine (小肠)	Taiyang Small Intestine Meridian of Hand (手太阳小肠经)
15:00 - 17:00	shēn shí	申時	Urinary Bladder (膀胱)	Taiyang Bladder Meridian of Foot (足太阳膀胱经)
17:00 - 19:00	yǒu shí	酉時	Kidney (肾)	Shaoyin Kidney Meridian of Foot (足少阴肾经)
19:00 - 21:00	xū shí	戌時	Pericardium (心包)	Jueyin Pericardium Meridian of Hand (手厥阴心包经)
21:00 - 23:00	hài shí	亥時	San jiao (三焦)	Shaoyang Sanjiao Meridian of Hand (手少阳三焦经)

The 12 Primary Meridians Channelling Time-table

The table above outlines the flow order of the 12 principal meridians and their corresponding active periods throughout the day.

Application of Meridian-Collateral System Theory

In the Earth's weather system, the movement of heat energy between the Earth's water bodies, land mass, and atmosphere through local and global ocean currents, affects the regulation of local weather conditions.

Similarly, when some parts of our body are not well, different sensations will be felt at a distance along the Meridian-Collateral System. When a part of the human body is stimulated through this system, this stimulation will channelled into the relative organ visceral in the body, thereby inducing relative changes either physiologically or pathologically.

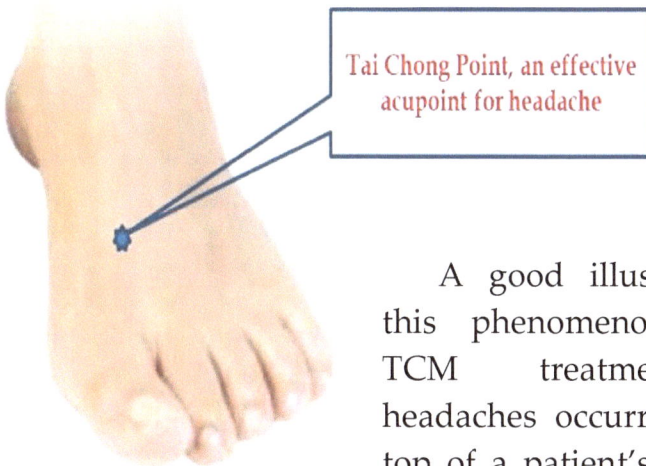

Tai Chong Point, an effective acupoint for headache

A good illustration of this phenomenon is the TCM treatment for headaches occurring at the top of a patient's head. An effective acupoint to alleviate the symptom occurs at the side of our big toe, the Tai Chong 太冲 (LV3), a point in the Jueying Liver Meridian of the foot.

Treatment Fundamental

The functional activities of our internal organs and pathological changes may also be transmitted to the body surface via the meridian system, manifesting themselves through different signs and symptoms. A feeling of numbness is associated with poor circulation of Qi within the meridian-collateral system, while a sharp pain is associated with blockages of Qi flow through the systems. Through the "Syndrome Differentiation" diagnostic approach, TCM practitioners are able to administer appropriate acupuncture treatments. The patient will then experience sensations such as soreness and tightness along the meridian, indicating the "arrival of Qi" and "induction of Qi" which activates the self-healing mechanisms in the body.

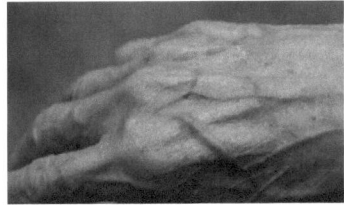

Regulating Body's Balance

Where there is disharmony of Qi -blood and excess or deficiency of Yin or Yang in our body, acupuncture treatments can be used to trigger regulatory actions of the meridian system by reducing what is excessive, or reinforcing what is deficient to regulate the body and maintain its equilibrium.

For example, when the stomach is functioning poorly, a mild stimulation given at the acupoint associated with the stomach may strengthen gastric contraction and increase the concentration of gastric juice. As the stomach is in a hyperactive state, a strong stimulation will cause an inhibitory effect. A typical acupoint used in such situations is the Zusanli 足三里 (ST 36) point of the Yangming Stomach Meridian of the foot, which through acupressure manipulations, can regulate peristalsis and secreting functions of the stomach.

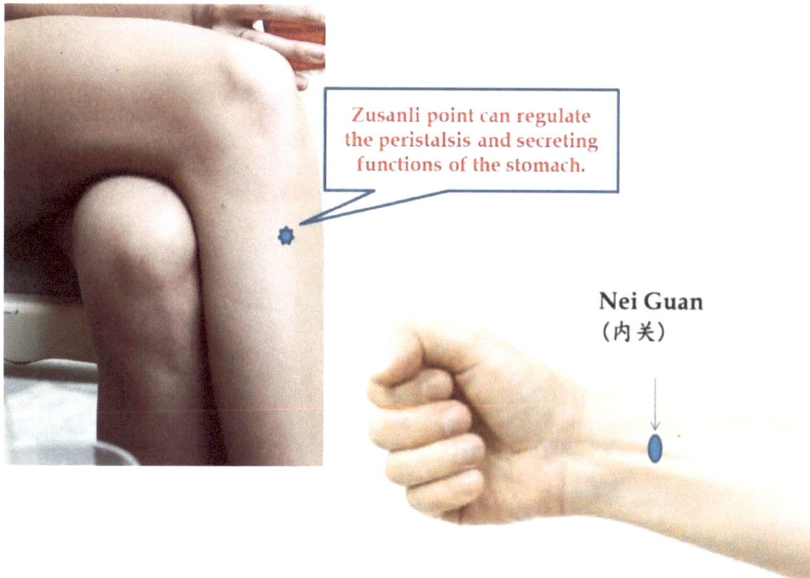

Zusanli point can regulate the peristalsis and secreting functions of the stomach.

Nei Guan
（内关）

Those experiencing palpitations and discomfort in the chest area may apply acupressure on Neiguan 内关 (PC 6), a point of the Jueyin Pericardium Meridian of hand. This helps to regulate the sensation by increasing heartbeat and, in some conditions, inhibit heart throbbing. This is the benefit of dual regulation in keeping the balance in our body, a key component in acupuncture treatment.

Conclusion

Just as changes to the ocean currents and destruction to the flow the global ocean conveyer belts affect global climates, the next time when you feel blue or not in the right mood, you may consider seeking treatment to see whether your internal Qi flow along your body superhighway - the meridian-collateral systems - is at its optimal state.

Keep up with the flow

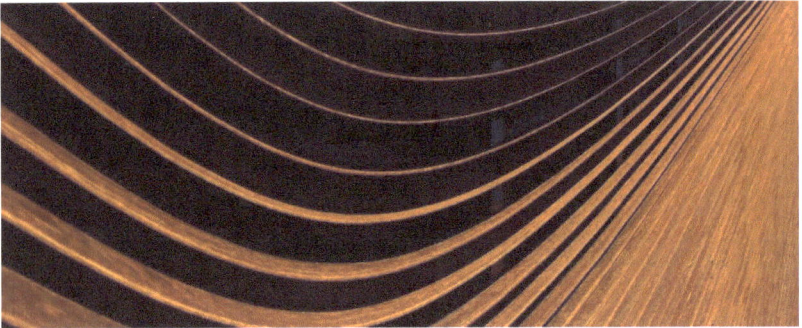

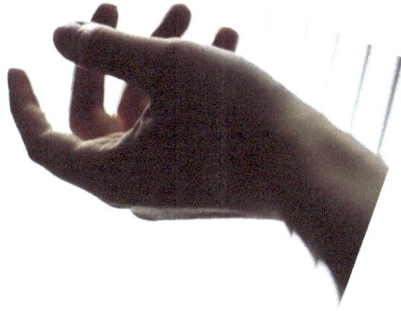

6. The Effective Acupoints To Good Health

In our previous chapter, we touched on the concept of Qi operating like a superhighway in your body, channelling energy and nutrients throughout your body. This chapter, I will show you how TCM identifies Acupoints and works along this superhighway to keep your body systems in balance, ensuring you are in the pink of health.

Chinese medicinal systems place close attention to individualised and targeted treatment based on the unique body constitution of an individual and how it interacts with the universe. In our previous chapter, we touched on the 365 acupuncture points within the body and their specific therapeutic profiles, which can be utilised during acupuncture or tuina/ acupressure massage

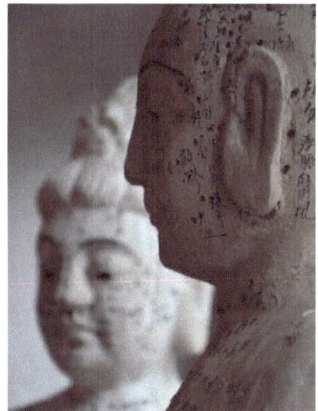

treatments. Here I will show you how to keep healthy by mastering **seven** important acupoints. By choosing one or two of these seven effective acupoints to massage a couple of minutes each day – making it part of your daily routine – you will maintain good health for a long time to come.

The Unique Body's Dimension Measurement System

Acupressure massage is a non-invasive manipulation technique that helps to balance the body's conditions. It activates your body meridians by improving circulation and enhance your well-being. Before I share with you the seven effective acupoints that you can use for health maintenance, let me show you how we determine these points around our body using the "Unique Body's Dimension Measurement" concept. Utilising a measurement unit known as **Cun (寸)**, TCM's "Body's Length Dimension Measurement" system can locate acupoints easily and accurately while accommodating to each individual's shape and size. A Cun is an individualised unit belonging uniquely to you.

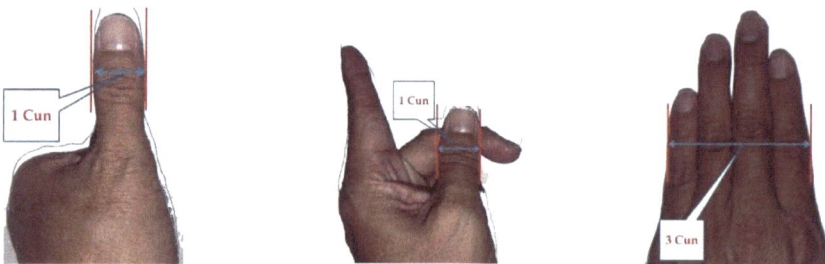

Author's hands Cun units

The system uses a simple approach to determine 1 **Cun** and 3 **Cun**. 1 Cun corresponds to the width of your thumb, and the width of the two crests of your middle finger. If you bend your middle finger, and place your finger on it, you will notice that the width of your thumb is exactly equal to the width of the two crests of your middle finger. 3 **Cun** corresponds to the width of the four fingers placed close to each other.

The system further dictates that different parts of the body have its corresponding Cun length which is unique to each individual. For example the distance between the wrist crease and the elbow crease is **12 Cun** and the distance between the two nipples is **8 Cun**, and the distance between the depressions on the outer side of the knee to the tip of the outer ankle is **16 Cun**.

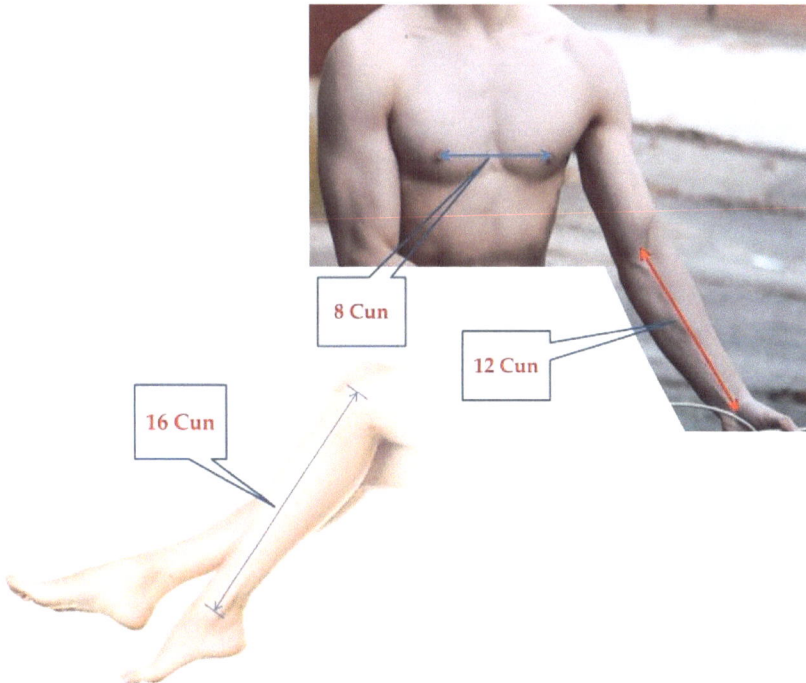

The Seven Acupoints

With an understanding of how to locate the acupoint on our body, let's look into the seven effective acupoints for general health maintenance; they are:

- **Nei Guan(内关),**

- **He Gu (合谷),**

- **Tai Xi(太溪),**

- **ZuSanli (足三里),**

- **SanYinJiao(三阴交),**

- **Guan Yuan (关元),**

- **Zhong Wan (中脘) .**

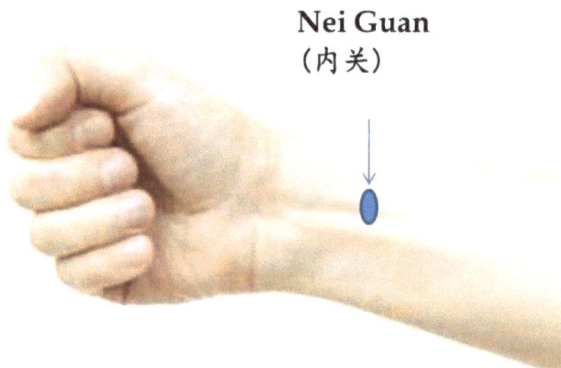

Nei Guan
(内关)

Nei Guan(内 关) acupoint belongs to the Pericardium Meridian and is located on the inner-side of the forearm, 2 Cun above to the wrist crease, in between the 2 tendons (the tendons of palmaris longus and flexor carpi radialis).

Nei Guan(内关) acupoint is known to be the protective umbrella of the heart, and is commonly used to address symptoms associated with Heart diseases, such as rheumatic heart disease, myocarditis, coronary heart disease. It helps prevent myocardial infarction and heart attack. It has the therapeutic effect of relieving chest tightness, regulating the heart, calming and alleviating nausea and vomiting.

Massaging technique: Press the acupoint of your left hand with your left thumb. Slowly rotate the your left wrist, about 30 times, when you find a sore sensation,

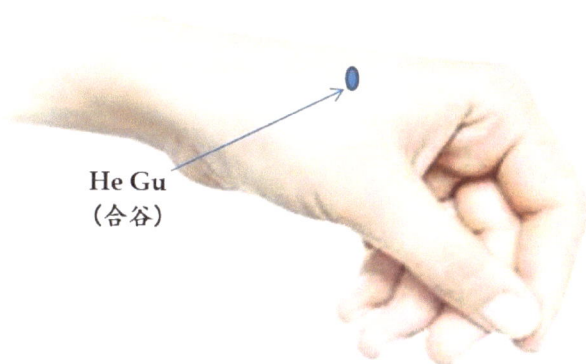

He Gu
(合谷)

He Gu (合谷) acupoint belongs to the Large Intestine Meridian. It is located at the back of the palm, on the dorsum of the hand, approximately at the midpoint of the second metacarpal bone.

This is the most common acupoint for natural therapeutic pain management, regardless of injury or medical diseases and also use in treatment for dizziness, nausea, and other abnormal symptoms.

Massaging this acupoint will help strengthen your Defensive Qi, restoring the Yang Qi and nourish the facial muscle group. However, for pregnant lady, this point should be avoided as it helps to induce labour.

Massaging technique: Press this acupoint with your thumb at the midpoint of the second metacarpal bone, about 50 times each, with slightly heavier strength, when press there is a tingling feeling.

For treatment related to facial muscle group, alternate the hand being manipulated, that is, right hand for the left side of the face, vice versa

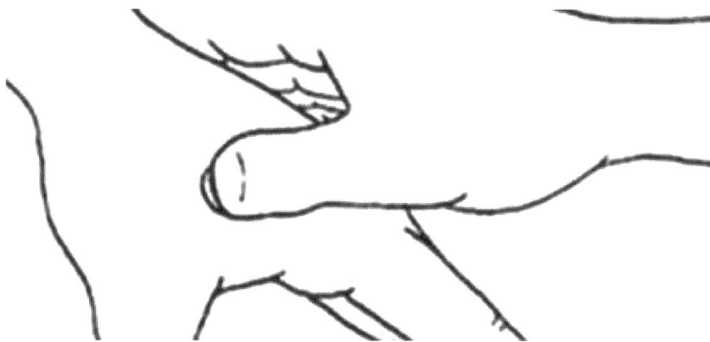

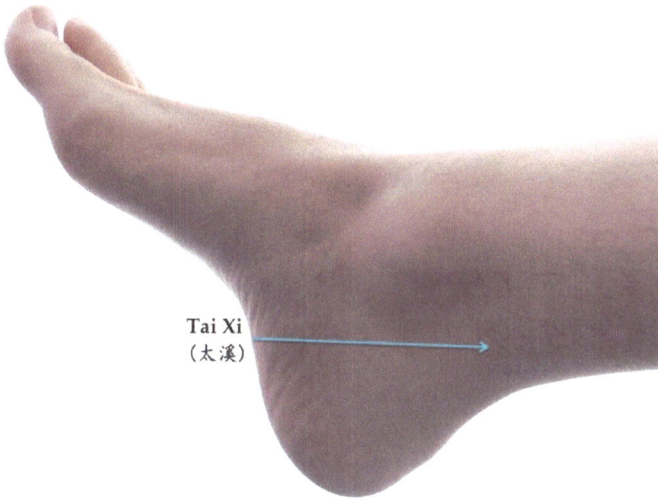

Tai Xi(太 溪) acupoint belongs to the kidney Meridian and is located behind the ankle, at the midpoint between the tip of the ankle and the calcaneal tendon. It is the choice acupoint for chronic kidney diseases, such as chronic renal failure, diabetes, kidney and oedema, weak legs, and backache.

Massaging this acupoint helps to nourishes kidney Yin, strengthen kidney Yang, and the lumbar spine.

Massaging Technique: Rub this acupoint with 3 middle fingers starting from behind the ankle using an upward movement for about 50 times each. You should feel a tingling sensation at the middle of the base of the foot.

Zu San Li
(足三里)

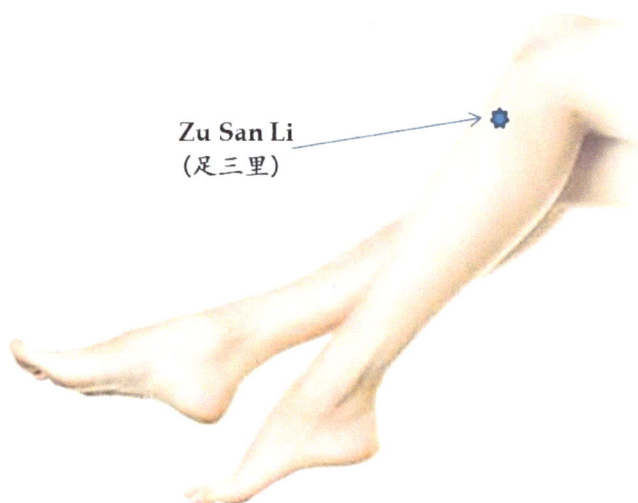

ZuSanli (足三里) acupoint is located on the leg, one Cun lateral to the tibia's anterior crest, and 3 Cun below the depression to the lateral side of the patella.

This acupoint is very effective for Qi nourishment and is known to have similar effects as ginseng.

It was commonly used for symptoms associated with sub-health conditions such as dizziness, chronic fatigue, anaemia caused by malnutrition, post-natal symptoms and for treatment for chronic diseases such as hypertension, diabetics.

Massaging Technique: It was recommend massaging on this point every day, by gently pressing and hitting the acupoint at any interval is useful for general health maintenance, as it can help to

Strengthens the Primordial Qi, Nourishes the blood and has a calming effect.

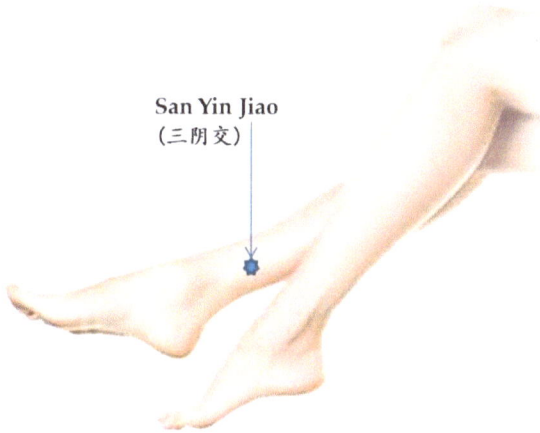

San Yin Jiao
(三阴交)

SanYinJiao (三阴交) acupoint is located 3 Cun directly above the tip of the inner ankle and slightly behind the tibia, also known as the Three Yin Intersection. The point where the Spleen, Kidney and Liver Yin meridian of the foot intersect.

This acupoint is a very effective for strengthening the spleen and nourishing the liver and kidney visceral systems. Massaging this point helps improve the transformation of the Spleen Visceral System, it also regulates blood, harmonise hormonal changes and eliminates stasis.

Massaging Technique: Massage this point daily by gently pressing or holding on to the point using one thumb and gently rotate the ankle.

Zhong Wan (中脘) acupoint belongs to the Conception meridian, and is located in the upper umbilical region, on the anterior midline, 4 Cun above the belly button.

This is an important acupoint for treating symptoms related to digestive systems. **Zhong Wan (中脘) acupoint where** the Conception **Qi,** the Lung Qi, the Spleen Qi, the Stomach Qi, and Triple Energizer meridians congregate.

Manipulating this acupoint will help to regulate symptoms associated with these meridians. This helps strengthen the stomach, calming and regulates the body's overall Qi dynamics.

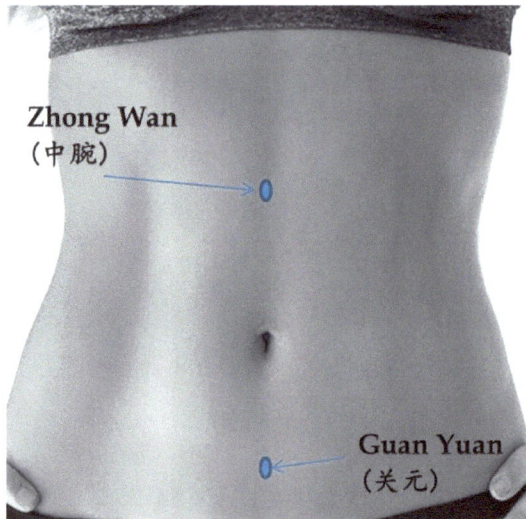

Guan Yuan (关元) acupoint belongs to the Conception meridian. It is located in the pubic region, on the anterior midline, 3 Cun below the belly button.

This acupoint is key in restoring youthful vitality. It is particularly effective for treating infertility, impotence, irregular menstruation, and other symptoms associated with reproductive system and Prostate related syndrome.

Massaging this acupoint can strengthens Primordial Qi, strengthens and nourishes the Kidney visceral system, help address prolapses.

Massaging Technique: Use 3 middle fingers to gently massage this acupoint in clockwise rotation for 1-2 minutes, followed by counter-clockwise rotation for another 1-2 minutes, and stop when local area feels warm.

The above mentioned seven effective acupoints for general health maintenance are commonly being adopted by TCM practitioners in their treatments. Besides striving for a healthy diet regime, as a simple guideline, if we can massage one or two of these acupoints daily, it goes a long way in helping us to maintain healthy living too.

A **5 minutes massage session per day is more effective than a 45 minutes weekly SPA/ massage session.**

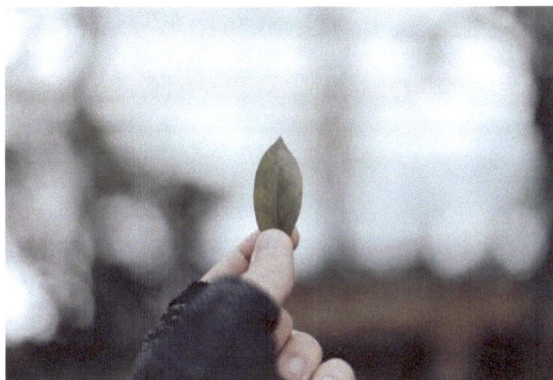

7. You Are Unique!

In this chapter, I show you how TCM evaluates different body constitutions and how you as an individual will be able to identify ways to identify your unique and personalised health profile.

The concept of body constitution differentiation is widely used in TCM practice. Throughout its development, different classification methods have been adopted: the Yin-Yang's constitution classification, the 5-elements' body constitution classification and body-syndrome classification, and the latest 9–body constitution classification developed by Professor Wang Qi from the Beijing University of TCM. These different classifications are indicative of the importance of constitutional consideration in TCM clinical diagnosis and treatment processes, laying the foundation for health promotion and disease prevention through diet management.

Body constitution varies from person to person. Whether its through genes inherited from our parents, or nourishment, upbringing or other influences acquired from our environment. Each one of us is unique due to the different structural, physiological and psychological aspects we faced during our growth. The unique body constitution of a person determines how we live and behave, as well as our susceptibility to pathogens and disease development.

According to Professor Wang Qi, our body constitution can be divided into nine types: neutral, Qi (blood) deficient, Yang deficient, Yin deficient, blood stasis, phlegm and dampness, damp-heat, Qi stagnation and special constitution. Generally, body constitution affects an individual's emotions and behaviour, and how they respond to causes of illness. Undesirable health conditions and illnesses arise when our bodies lose balance.

The Nine Types Of Body Constitution

1. Neutral

Individuals have a strong physique, stable emotional or mental state and feel optimistic. They often have lustrous complexion and hair, bright eyes, proper senses of smell and taste,

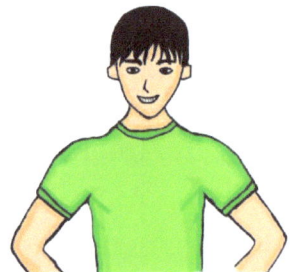

red and moist lips, resistance to fatigue, good sleep and appetite, normal bowel and urinary habits. They are adaptable to environmental changes.

Nutrition Diet recommendation: Eat a wide variety of foods and in moderation, always maintain a balanced diet and avoid foods that are too oily or spicy.

Health Tips: Exercise regularly, practicing Qigong, Yoga and meditation.

2. Qi (Blood) deficient

Individuals tend to have flabby muscles, are introverted and timid in personality. They often have a feeble voice, shortness of breath, fatigue, catching cold or flu easily, with sweating and teeth marks in the tongue margin. They are sensitive to environmental changes. Since these individuals are relatively weak in immune functions, it usually takes a longer time for them to recover from illnesses.

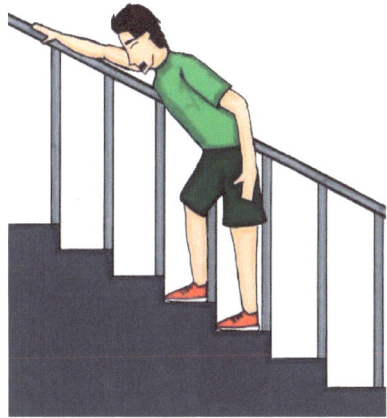

Nutrition Diet recommendation: Eat more foods that nourish Qi and spleen functions. Avoid foods that have a purging effect on the body's Qi.

Herbal medicines to consider:

中文	Latin Name	English Name	Hanyu Pinying
黄芪	Radix Astragali	Astragali	Huángqí
人参	Radix Ginseng	Ginseng	Rénshēn
当归	Radix Angelicae Sinensis	Angelica	Dāngguī

3. Yang deficient

Individuals tend to have flabby muscles, are quiet and introverted in personality. They often complain about cold hands and feet, cold feeling in the stomach, are sensitive to low temperatures or noises, sleepiness, discomfort after eating cold foods, and a pale and bulky tongue. They often feel uncomfortable in windy, cold and humid environments. They are susceptible to health problems such as low core energy, lower libido, diarrhoea anxiety, panic attacks and fear.

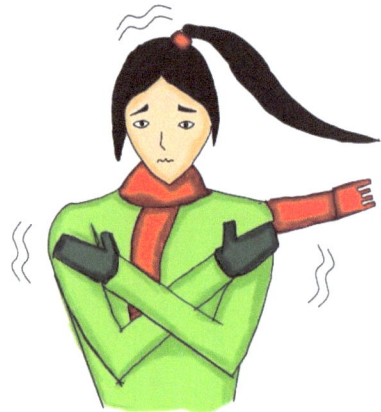

Nutrition Diet recommendation: Eat more foods that have warming characteristics. Eat less foods that are raw and considered cold in nature.

Herbal medicines to consider:

中文	Latin Name	English Name	Hanyu Pinying
鹿茸	Ccornu Cervi Pantotrichum	Pilose Antler	Lù róng
巴戟天	Radix Morindae Officinalis	Morinda Root	Bā jǐ tiān
杜仲	Cortex Eucommiae	Eucommia Bark	Dù zhòng
肉苁蓉	Herba Cistanches	Cistanche Deserticola	Ròu cōng róng

4. Yin deficient

Individuals usually have a thin physique, are outgoing and impatient in personality. They like to complain about warm palms and soles, mouth dryness and dry nose. They have preference for cold drinks and often feel uncomfortable in hot and dry environments. They are susceptible to cough, fatigue, seminal emissions, dry stools, constipation, insomnia and some chronic conditions.

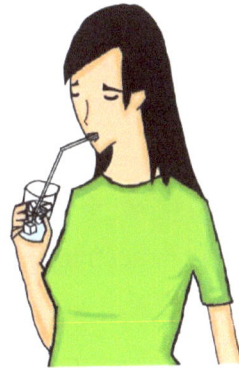

The Nutrition Diet recommendation: Eat more foods that are yin nourishing or help in generating fluids in the body. Eat less foods that have warming and/or diuretic properties.

Herbal medicines to consider:

中文	Latin Name	English Name	Hanyu Pinying
麦冬	Radix Ophiopogonis	Dwarf Lilyturf Tuber	Mài dōng
石斛	Herba Dendrobii	Dendrobium	Shí hú
女贞子	Fructus Ligustri Lucidi	Glossy Privet Fruit	Nǚ zhēn zi
黄精	Polygonatum sibiricum	Polygonatum	Huáng jīng

5. Phlegm and dampness

Individuals are usually over weight and have a tummy. They are mild, and have steady and patient personalities. They often have an oily face, sticky or sweet taste in the mouth, excessive throat secretions, sweating, chest stuffiness, preference for sweet and greasy foods, and a thick tongue coating. They often feel uncomfortable in humid and rainy environments. They are susceptible to diabetes, metabolic syndrome or cardiovascular diseases.

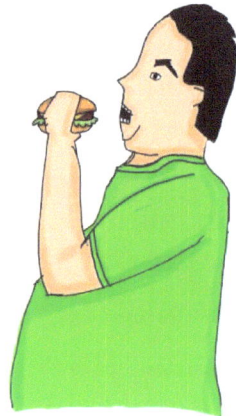

Nutrition Diet recommendation: Maintain a bland and balanced diet. Eat more foods that help improve urination and purge dampness from the body. Eat less foods that are sweet, stodgy and greasy.

Herbal medicines to consider:

中文	Latin Name	English Name	Hanyu Pinying
生姜	Rhizoma Zingiberis Recens	Fresh Ginger	Shēng jiāng
茯苓	Poria	Poria	Fú líng
冬瓜皮	Exocarpium Benincasae	Chinese waxgourd peel	Dōngguā pí
瞿麦	Herba Dianthi	lilac pink herb	Qú mài
薏苡仁	Semen Coicis	Coix Seed	Yì yǐ rén

6. Damp-heat

Individuals have either a normal or thin physique. They tend to be irritable and short-tempered. They often have an oily face that erupts with acne or pimples, a bitter or strong taste in the mouth, fatigue or heaviness of the body, a feeling of incompletion after defecation, dry stools, yellow urine, excess vaginal discharge in females, wet scrota in males, and a yellow and greasy tongue coating. They are sensitive to humid and hot environments especially in

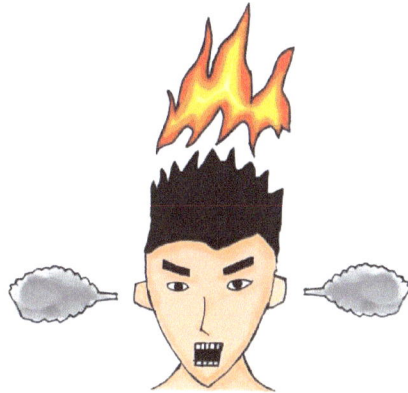

late summer or early autumn. They are susceptible to skin problems and urinary difficulties.

Nutrition Diet recommendation: Eat more foods that help to cleanse heat and dampness from the body. Eat less foods that are heaty, astringent and oily.

Herbal medicines to consider:

中文	Latin Name	English Name	Hanyu Pinying
地肤子	Fructus Kochiae	Belvedere Fruit	Dì fū zi
茵陈	Herba Artemisiae Scopariae	Virgate Wormwood Herb	Yīn chén
金钱草	Herba Lysimachiae	Loosestrife	Jīn qián cǎo
黄连	Rhizoma Coptidis	Coptis	Huáng lián

7. Blood stasis

Individuals tend to be impatient and forgetful. They often have a dull complexion, spots on the face, dark-red lips, dark circles under eyes, lacklustre or rough skin, unknown bruises on the body surface, and varicose veins. They often feel uncomfortable in cold environments. They are susceptible to bleeding, painful conditions and abnormal growths.

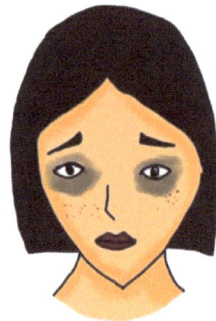

Nutrition Diet recommendation: Eat more foods that help promote blood circulation. Eat less foods that are oily in nature.

Herbal medicines to consider:

中文	Latin Name	English Name	Hanyu Pinying
三七	Radix Notoginseng	Notoginseng	Sān qī
益母草	Herba Leonuri	Motherwort Herb	Yì mǔ cǎo
红花	Stigma Croci	Saffron	Hóng huā
丹参	Radix Salviae Miltiorrhizae	Salvia	Dān shēn

8. Qi stagnation

Individuals are mostly thin and tend to be emotionally unstable, melancholic or suspicious. They often have a depressed mood, are nervous, anxious, timid, sigh frequently and have heart palpitations. They respond relatively poorly to stressful situations, especially in winter, autumn and rainy days. They are susceptible to insomnia, depression, anxiety disorder and breast lumps.

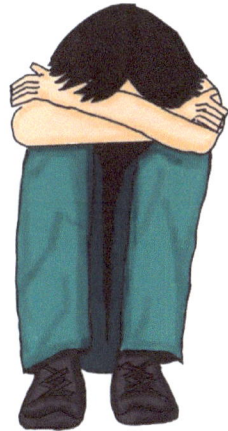

Nutrition Diet recommendation: Eat more foods that help disperse Qi, remove stagnation, improve digestion and provide calming effects.

Herbal medicines to consider:

中文	Latin Name	English Name	Hanyu Pinying
柴胡	Radix Bupleuri	Chinese Thorowax Root	Chái hú
川芎	Herba Leonuri	Turmeric	Chuān xiōng
郁金	Radix Curcumae	Saffron	Yù jīn
陈皮	Pericarpium Citri Reticulatae	Dried Tangerine Peel	Chén pí

9. Special or sensitive

Individuals usually have inborn weakness. They are very sensitive to drugs, foods, smells, pollen or other environmental allergens. They are prone to sneezing, runny nose, panting, and often develop nasal congestion, wheals, itchiness and even purple spots or patches under the skin. Common health problems among individuals are drug allergies, hay fever, eczema and asthma. They respond relatively poorly to external influences, and their health problems

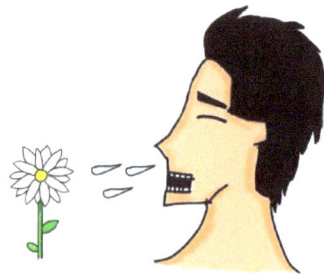

can easily be induced by seasonal changes.

Nutrition Diet recommendation: Maintain a balanced diet. Avoid foods that may trigger the onset of the sensitivity. Eat less foods that are spicy or those considered to have simulative effects, such as buckwheat, crab and prawns etc.

Conclusion

In reality, it is difficult to classify individuals to one particular body constitution type, as everyone will manifest a mixture of conditions. For example, Yin deficiency and damp-heat; Qi deficiency and dampness; Qi stagnation and blood stasis. In such cases, you may want to consider consulting a TCM practitioner to give you a diagnosis to determine your individualized body constitution. This is similar to an annual health check report that allows you to make informed decisions regarding what you should be eating for your next meal.

In addition, your body constitution is not constant nor unchangeable. Factors such as the environment we live in, our mental state, our diet routines, our daily activities and diseases can easily change the body's condition. **Taking control of your health according to the body constitution types is an important aspect of health maintenance.**

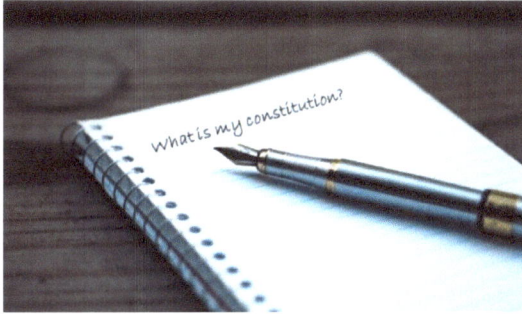

8. 7 Minutes to know your body types

The following set of questions - 40 questions – allows you to gain a preliminary understanding of your body constitution type. These dichotomous questions have been designed to let you to reflect upon experiences and feelings which you have in the immediate-past 12 months.

As you go through the questionnaire, which takes about 7 minutes, you may have some questions, or you may feel that the descriptions are look strange or foreign, please just ignore it. Although you may not have such experiences, but others may have.

Circle the number representing questions related to your personal experiences and feelings. Populate your selection into the table at the end of questionnaire.

If you circle 3 or more numbers in each row, then you are likely to belong to this body constitution. If you circle 2 numbers then you may be inclined to belong to this constitution, yet still can be considered having a normal, healthy constitution.

BODY CONSTITUTION SELF-CHECK

Based on your last 12 Month's experience and feeling, answer the following questions:

1 Feel shortness of breath easily.
2 Mouth often feels bitter, bad breath or odour.
3 Often have dry stool.
4 Often feel pain on the breasts or along the rip area.
5 Often have loose stool, clear urine colour and abundant volume.
6 Often feel heavy in the body and limbs.
7 The eyes often have red lining.
8 Allergy to medicines, foods, odours, changes of weather.
9 Prefers to stay quiet, often speaks with a low, frail voice.
10 Face and tip of the nose look oily and shiny, prone to acne.
11 Palms, soles and chest area often feel feverish.
12 Sentimental, emotionally frail easily frightened.
13 Often have cold limbs.
14 Palms and soles often sweaty and wet.
15 Skin bruises easily, the gums bleed easily
16 Often have stuffy nose, sneezing, runny nose, or even asthma, even when not having flu.
17 Often feel tired and weak.
18 Often have sticky stool.
19 Hot Flushes
20 Often feel depressed, low mood and sigh for no apparent reason.
21 Stomach area often feels cold.
22 Often noticed swelling eyes.
23 Vulnerable to experience variety of pains.

24 Vulnerable to get rashes.
25 Vulnerable to cold.
26 Urine feels hot, urine colour often yellowish.
27 Dry eyes.
28 Easily tensed, flustered, palpitation, anxious, insomnia.
29 Wear more clothes than others
30 Usually have lots of phlegm.
31 Dark complexion or pigmentation , dark eye areas.
32 Skin often shows red scratches.
33 Often perspires.
34 Women have yellowish vaginal discharge/ men's scrotum often wet.
35 Often have dry mouth and throat.
36 Throat often has clogging sensation.
37 Feel uncomfortable after drinking cooling stuff.
38 Mouth often feels sticky or sweet.
39 Dry, rough skin.
40 Blood spots often appears on the skin, due to allergies.

Analysis of Body Types:

1	9	17	25	33	Qi deficient
2	10	18	26	34	Damp heat
3	11	19	27	35	Yin deficient
4	12	20	28	36	Qi stagnant
5	13	21	29	37	Yang deficient
6	14	22	30	38	Phlegm damp
7	15	23	31	39	Blood stasis
8	16	24	32	40	Special/Sensitive

Now that you have completed your self-assessment, if you belong to a specific type, you can consult the previous chapter for associated nutrition guidance. You may also take a step further to apply the acupoint massaging techniques. Bear in mind that since you are doing this based solely on this book, there is limitations to the assessment. Do consult an expert.

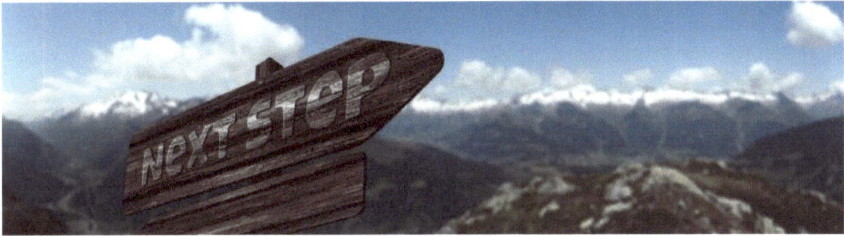

9. Next Step

We have come to the first milestone of our learning journey. I trust that you have gained much insight into the wisdom of TCM.

Perhaps, you want to take a step further and want to explore further how TCM can maintain your personal health even better. I have developed courses and workshops on TCM for people like you, who want more in-depth understanding and benefit from it. I list the courses that I have been conducting.

TCM Inspired Management & Leadership Programme

- A Healthy leader - A Great Company
- The 5 Elements Approach to Corporate Management
- The Yin & Yang of leading in the Disruptive World

Singapore SkillsFuture Approved courses

- Professional Paediatric Massage
- TCM Disease Management
- Health through TCM for Senior
- Acupressure Massage Fundamental /Intermediate
- TCM Herbal Diet Fundamental /Intermediate

- TCM Treatment for Children & Youth
- TCM for Men

Online courses @ Udemy

- How to perform Effective TCM Baby & Child Massage
- Why am I fat when I don't eat much! - How TCM helps!
- Professional Paediatric Massage

I am in the process of writing the following books. I look forward to share them with you soonest possible.

TCM Herbal Diet – Eat for wellness

As Hippocrates said "Let thy food be thy medicine!" I will discuss the use of food as medicine through TCM medicated or herbal diet. You will learn individual constitutions of such diets and the impact of geographical environment and the influence of seasonal changes. You will learn how a proper choice of diet can go a long way in maintaining your health.

TCM Treatment for Children and Youth

TCM treatment for children and youth has been practised for thousands of years. I will introduce you to the physiological characteristics of infants and children, common illnesses associate with them, methods of diagnosis, treatment and prevention in TCM. You will learn the use of common Chinese medicine for your daily diet and TCM Paediatric Massage techniques.

The Magical Touch – Acupressure Massage

Massage, the sense of touch, is not just for comforting and pampering ourselves. Besides maintaining general health, massage provides significant relief for those suffer from chronic pain or long-term illnesses. Enhance your massage knowledge by understanding TCM meridian theory and proper acupressure techniques.

In the meantime, please take sometimes to reflect upon what you have learnt and the next steps in your personal journey to health. I encourage you to visit my Facebook page at **https://www.facebook.com/tcmandyou** and click like to stay connected.

I look forward to partnering with you on your journey to greater health.

Disclaimer

While every detail and evidence with respect to the value of TCM and the effectiveness of such methods and techniques have been carefully studied, the advice and information contained in this Book is and purely introductory. This book neither purports, nor is intended, to be advice on a particular illness or disease or health issue. No reader should act on the basis of anything contained in the book without seeking independent professional medical advice. No responsibility or liability whatsoever can be accepted by the author, for any loss, damage or injury that may arise from any person acting on any advice or information contained in this book and all such liabilities are expressly disclaimed.

Reflection:

Thank you for taking time to read the book. Please spend some time to reflect upon how TCM can play a part in your journey toward healthy living. You can send your thoughts to: reflection101@tcmandyou.com

www.ingramcontent.com/pod-product-compliance
Lightning Source LLC
Chambersburg PA
CBHW041711200326
41518CB00001B/150